I Don't Know How Long My Short-Term Memory Is . . .

Feldenkrais Method® and BrainEase

I Don't Know How Long My Short-Term Memory Is . . .

Feldenkrais Method® and BrainEase

Nancy Haller

Second Edition
Printed in the United States by
Lifetime Connections Publishing

Third Edition Published 2023
Second Edition Published 2020
Original Edition Published 2012
Printed in the United States by
Lifetime Connections Publishing

Library of Congress Number – 2012946702

ISBN-13: 978-0-9881792-6-4 Paperback
ISBN-13: 978-0-9881792-5-7 E-Book

©2010, 2012, 2015, 2020, 2023 by Nancy Haller

All rights reserved. No part of this publication may be reproduced, stored in a retrieval system, or transmitted, in any form or by any means, electronic, mechanical, photocopying, recording, or otherwise, without the prior written permission of the publisher.

I don't know how long my short-term memory is . . . is written by Nancy Haller and is not intended as medical advice. Its intent is solely informational and educational. Please consult a health professional should the need for one be indicated.

The terms Feldenkrais Method®, Feldenkrais®, Awareness Through Movement®, Functional Integration® and The Feldenkrais Guild® are Registered Marks of the Feldenkrais Guild of North America®.

Table of Contents

Begin the Conversation 7
Been There, Doing That 12
Part 1 19
People With Brain Issues 20
Types of Brain Issues 22
    Brain Injured 22
    Brain Fogged 24
    Brain Tired 26
Do You Know Someone 27
What's Happening? 28
Fear, Anger, Frustration 30
Where to Start 32
Memories 36
Attention Span 38
Family, Friends, and Others 40
Caretaker Burnout 44
Observations 48
Hearing 54
Rest 58
Sleep 60
Activities 62
School 66
Work 70
Retirement 72
Going Shopping 78
Travel 82
Getting Out of the House 86
Crossroads 88
Decisions and Choices 89
Food, Supplements, Alcohol, and Drugs 94
Environment 100
Image of Self 104
We Are Asymmetrical 106
Balance, Posture, and Movement 108
    Balance 109

Posture 112
Movement 114
Safety, Security, and Support 116
Part II Sharing the Keys.. 118
For the Rest of Your Life... 119
About the Feldenkrais Method® 121
Learn to Learn... 125
30 to 60 Second Moments of Awareness 139
First Things First.. 141
Who Will Benefit?.. 147
Strategies For Success 148
1. Weight Through the Heels... 151
2. Feet to Head 153
3. Feet Observing 155
4. Breathing... 157
5. Head toward the Ceiling 161
6. Feet to Hips 163
7. Heel to Toe 165
8. Attention to One Side 167
9. Circles with the Nose... 169
10. Eyes in the Back of Head... 171
11. Straight Arms Swinging 173
12. Balancing a Quarter on the Head................................... 175
13. Laughing Daily 177
14. Nose to Neck... 179
15. Swinging Arms—One Hand Pushing.............................. 181
16. Moving from Sitting to Standing 183
17. Tongue Between the Teeth 185
18. Finger Pressing, One at a Time...................................... 187
19. Building a Brain White Board or Screen 189
20. Step Backwards 191
21. Open Your Eyes.. 195
22. Walking with Open Eyes 199
23. Climbing the Stairs 201
24. Balancing on One Leg 203
25. Chewing... 205
26. Rocking the Pelvis 207

27. Rolling the Feet 209
28. Grip—Move from Large to Small 211
29. Move the Top of the Neck 215
30. Move from the Bottom of the Neck................217
31. Imagine 219
Just a Few of the Resources in America...............223
Add Your Favorites 225
Dedication and Huge Gratitude 226

Laugh...

At yourself,
With yourself,
and
For yourself.

It is all okay!

(**Sometimes,** my short-term memory is conveniently
very,

very,

very

SHORT!)

Begin the Conversation

Are you living with some form of brain injury--concussion, stroke, TIA, dementia, Alzheimer's, TBI (traumatic brain injury), brain damage, disease, or degeneration?

Are you experiencing brain fog, raging hormonal imbalance, aging brain, drug dependency, alcohol dependency, environmental toxicity, or chronic pain?

Are you totally brain tired--feeling like you are exhausted, totally overloaded, overwhelmed, over stressed and over it?

Do you know someone who is experiencing any of these issues to some degree or another? This book is for people who are working with someone or people who are experiencing brain issues as a helpful tool to clarify and address some of the problems and processes that continue to occur daily.
This book is for YOU!

Feel free to read this book a page or a chapter at a time.

Read it in whatever way is most comfortable for you. Put it down when you need a break. Pick it up when you are ready to receive more information.

There are blank pages throughout the book. These allow the opportunity to stop, rest, and enjoy a space of nothing-ness.

Two parts make up this conversation

The first part of this book describes common situations that occur in daily life. The examples offer the opportunity to assess yourself and your personal relationship with family, friends, and people in your community. Everyone, as they progress through their lives, will be touched these issues. People of all ages, from children to seniors, experience these difficulties as they face new brain challenges presented every day. The fear of being a failure, inept, an invalid, or disabled, makes this conversation delicate.

The second part of this book consists of **thirty-one individual 30- to 60-second "moments of awareness."** Each of the simple short exercises designed to increase attention to small details in movement. These small movement sequences focus the brain to awareness of different areas of the body. As awareness grows, the image of our personal self grows clear.

Neuroplasticity is when the brain creates new pathways; thereby creating memories. Focusing on how small details tie together will allow the process of replicating action easier.

With Brain issues, communication to and from the brain takes longer. Information presented in an understandable form is processed and filed for future use. This allows various degrees of development, which continue from birth to death throughout all of life.

Only in hindsight, can I assess walking through life without the information needed to understand how all the pieces would fit into the whole picture. The synchronistic process of layering events assisted my educational process, resulting in acquiring the necessary assessment skills to observe my brain in terms of strength and weakness.

It appears that finding language to explain situations and articulate details and experiences from the brain-injured point of view is a very unusual skill. While many experts are extremely knowledgeable in how the brain functions, they lack the personal experience of living with brain issues. My education and proficiency offer rare opportunities to look at both sides of brain issues. As I walk into my future, by working with teams of experts and brain-issue survivors, together we can develop materials and tools to improve healing outcomes for many who are facing their own brain injuries.

Begin with one exercise—incorporate it into your daily life. Add another exercise, as you are comfortable. There is no particular order—choose an exercise you find interesting.

Each day is a treasure . . .

Find the gems!

Been There, Doing That

One of the last things I thought I would ever hear . . .

"You do know you have a brain injury . . ."

The truth . . . I did not.

Synchronicity in life is an amazing thing.

It is with hindsight that I now assess how I walked each step in my life without the information needed to understand how all the pieces would fit into the whole picture. My time and life been a synchronistic process of layered events that assisted in my educational process. This process resulted in acquiring necessary assessment skills. Being able to observe my brain in terms of where I am strong and where there are weak areas is a rare skill few possess. Finding language to articulate details and experiences or explain situations from the brain-injured point of view is a very unusual skill. There are experts extremely knowledgeable in how the brain functions but they lack personal experience living with brain issues. My education and skills offer rare opportunities to look at both sides of these issues. Working with teams of experts and brain-issue survivors to develop materials and tools will improve the potential healing outcomes for many.

I began studying the somatic, mind and body connections when I joined Guild Certified Feldenkrais training in 1993, 7 years before my brain injury. Moshe Feldenkrais, D.Sc. developed the Feldenkrais Method® of somatic movement, in the mid-1940s. His method educates the mind through awareness of slow small movements that clarify posture, balance, and movement. The slow pace and light pressure allow the nervous system and brain time to receive the request and respond. These responses are necessary to change a pattern of restriction or injury. Through this re-education process, the body is able to replicate the newly learned patterns. Training in the method over four years, learning hundreds of movements and building self-awareness, changed my outlook and set the stage for the future.

Six years later, I suffered neurological damage while having jaw surgery. Although I looked the same, my brain was different. In the middle of the forest, I could not see the trees. Unaware of my injury, I immediately forged ahead in my life. I was a single parent raising two children, both on target for college. Familial and work obligations became my driving force in moving forward.

Between the recovery from surgery and the anesthesia fog, I assumed that my new condition of living in the "brain blue-screen" was relatively normal. I visually saw a shade of blue in my mind when I wanted to access something that was not available at the time. Sometimes it took me longer to remember something and other times I was unable to remember at all. I assumed the sorting and reconstruction of the lost files from my memory would occur over time. Some files are gone forever; both my long- and short-term memories were disrupted. I noticed changes in my balance and vision that varied depending on my activity and exhaustion levels. Some of the changes were just fleeting moments or stumbles in the path. To someone else observing me, they might not have been noticeable, but to me they were monumental. However, other things changed that I did not notice, and the difference to others was enormous.

Most noticeable to those around me was the change in my speech. When I spoke, it was with what sounded like a foreign accent. Everyone asked me, "Where are you from?" "Seattle," I replied, much to the confusion of everyone around me. I did not hear the accent or the change in my speech patterns. I continued to hear what I knew as my voice prior to the surgery.

In 2002, two years after surgery, I went to Deanna Britton, a speech therapist, she diagnosed me with Pseudo Foreign Accent Syndrome (FAS). FAS is a very rare speech disorder, with fewer than 100 people in the world having this diagnosis. FAS most commonly follows some form of brain injury or damage. The speakers sound like they have accents from another country. It is common to have speaking rhythm, word order, and sentence structure altered.

Upon further testing, my outcome stated I had only 52% of my individual word comprehension and 70% of my conversational sentences were understandable by others. My next step was a referral to a neurologist for further testing to look for a brain tumor or lesion.

I drove home from the appointment on auto-pilot. I was shocked and overwhelmed with the new information. It was not a possibility. It was not true. I was too busy. I did not have a brain problem.

The first round of testing was inconclusive. It was almost a year later that I had the scans read by another specialist. That was when I was informed that I had damage to several areas of my brain. Though I denied the information at first, I eventually faced to make an honest self-assessment.

My speech therapist explained that my brain now required more time to pass messages on to my mouth. This process can be likened to when someone is visiting a foreign country and looking to translate words. It takes longer to choose and then form words because one has to allow the brain this additional bit of time to formulate speech.

It was through my training in the brilliant work of Moshe Feldenkrais that I learned how to move slowly enough to find my way along this long, difficult road. The constant process of rehabilitation continues for me daily.

I was afraid to admit or acknowledge new changes and limitations that had become prominent. I questioned how people would perceive my experiencing brain fog or me, if they knew I had a brain injury or was brain tired. My work might be discounted, my ability to raise my family might be challenged, and my future might be dimmed by others' judgment. I worked tirelessly to hide all the difficulties, cover my shortcomings, and challenge myself to perform the seemingly impossible tasks that made up my life.

More than ten years later, I am still living with a brain injury. I personally experience being brain tired and suffering from brain fog. But I now realize that I am surrounded by a society of brain-tired people, and had been working with teens and aging family members who were living in brain fogs. These experiences were what stimulated my thoughts and brought this book to life. I share my insights, knowledge, and research in hopes that your path will be easier than mine. I have included thirty-one movement patterns to assist you in re-establishing the neuro-pathways in your brain.

Life moves forward regardless of the choices you make; it is important to look for great options.

Each day brings answers to my challenges and gratitude for the opportunities that are presented. I have a deep appreciation for the love, patience, and continued support received from those who surround me.

Tenacity has driven me to continue to live and work in this wonderful world every day. During this journey, I have maintained a Feldenkrais practice in the Seattle area, which I started in 1996. In 1999, one year before my surgery, I began my work with equestrians and horses across the country, which I continued after my surgery. From 1997 to 2004, I held the positions of President of the Feldenkrais Educational Foundation and Vice President of the Feldenkrais Guild of North America. I have been a national seminar presenter teaching continuing education courses in Neuromuscular Re-education and Medical Massage to massage and bodywork therapists since 2003. Both of my daughters have achieved graduate degrees in their respective fields. I completed my Master's degree in Somatic Movement Studies in 2010 from Lesley University. My thesis focused on a body of work, Neuromuscular Connections, developed to bridge the Feldenkrais Method and the massage community.

In 2011, I took the blood test for the MTHFR (Methylene Tetra Hydro Foliate Reductase) genetic mutation factor. My results were positive heterozygous for the A1298C MTHFR mutation. There are two different MTHFR mutations, C677T and A1298C. The list of possible conditions related to the C677T MTHFR mutation includes a propensity toward heart disease, stroke, high blood pressure, thrombosis, migraine headaches, glaucoma, psychiatric disorders and certain types of cancer.

Possible conditions related to the A1298C MTHFR mutation, the one I have, include a propensity toward headaches, seizures, insomnia, autism, fibromyalgia, ADD/ADHD, and chronic fatigue syndrome. More research information is now becoming available about this genetic factor and the challenges it puts on the neurological and physical systems. It affects the body's ability to tolerate drugs and other chemicals. It may have been a contributing factor to my brain injury during my surgery.

Almost ten years after my first appointment with Deanna Britton, the speech therapist, I scheduled an appointment for an assessment of the changes and similarities in my Foreign Accent Syndrome. Conversational sentence intelligibility had improved to 91% without conventional speech rehabilitation.

I attribute much of my improvement to use of the basic foundational theories Moshe Feldenkrais developed in his method, and an enormous spirit of tenacity.

I take each day one step at a time and each circumstance is assessed as it arises. I have acquired a great deal of patience and compassion for myself and for others.

No one will walk through this life unscathed.

I believe we come to the end of the road when we quit driving.

Part 1

People With Brain Issues

Every person will have brain issues at some point in their lifetime.

Join one of the largest groups in the world:
People With Brains . . .
and unfortunately . . . brain issues

Are you brain injured, brain tired or living in a brain fog?

Do you know anyone who is?

Are you a family member, friend, or member of the public sharing daily experiences with someone on the above list?

**You or someone you know could be recognized as a member of the group,
People with brain issues!!**

IF THERE WERE AN ORGANIZATION to be formed, it would internationally include everyone in the membership. Once people become aware of a change in their brain or a noticeable change occurred to someone they know, automatic eligibility to be become members of "People with Brain Issues" happens. This international membership would be created for the *brain injured, brain fogged or brain tired* and their friends, family and the rest of society. Everyone is welcome to participate in membership.

This membership has no structure, no board of directors, no staff, no policies, and no paperwork. There are no mandatory dues. There is no website, no newsletter, and no phone number to contact. There is no age limitation, no gender restriction, no educational background, no religion, and no race that is denied membership. No one has ever compiled a membership list.

Brain injury, brain fog and brain tiredness do not discriminate among those who are watching and anticipating personal inclusion at any moment.

When will you become a member?
Or have you already joined?

Look around.

You are not alone.

Types of brain issues

These are the four areas of discussion regarding brain issues

1. **Brain Injured**
2. **Brain Fogged**
3. **Brain Tired**
4. **Friends, Family and Others...Do you know someone?**

You can join one category or you can be included in multiple categories.

I have issues in all four areas with long standing acknowledgement.

There are four areas of people dealing with brain issues. Each person has similar needs for recognition and compassion. This is a book of strategies, ideas and observations to help people recognize and live with brain issues. Family, friends, and communities can acknowledge and assist with greater ease and understanding as they participate in the world with someone who is challenged.

Brain Injured

Brain injured people are medically diagnosed with certifiable brain damage or injury to any level or degree. This includes, but is not limited to, those who have experienced or are experiencing strokes, trauma, Traumatic Brain Injury (TBI), emotionally shocked brain, concussions, Post-Traumatic Stress Disorder (PTSD), neurological diseases, or shaken brain. These create injuries to the brain that affect our ability to function in our daily lives for long and short terms.

Brain injuries sometimes are not diagnosed for a variety of reasons. Small TBIs, minor concussions, or strokes may pass inspection until someone puts the puzzle together and requests further evaluation and testing.

There are many conditions that affect the brain and the ability to function in personal and public situations. Among these conditions are ADD/ADHD, autism, fibromyalgia, seizures, and a variety of autoimmune diseases. The list is long, and the mild-to-intense symptoms create constantly changing challenges on a daily basis.

Brain Fogged

Brain fog is an issue for people who have been under anesthesia or have undergone drug therapies. It may take a few months to a year or more for the brain to reconnect the circuits and pathways affected. Some may never fully recover. The person's initial health, age, and diagnosis, and the type of drugs and length of time taken, are factors which can impact the amount of damage incurred and the person's ability to recover.

Brain fog can also affect people diagnosed with chronic pain disorders like fibromyalgia or chronic fatigue syndrome, due to the distraction of constant pain.

Environmental toxicity and heavy metal exposure may also cause brain fog. We are not fully aware of all the invisible influences affecting the function of the brain.

Brain fog can also be a result of hormonal changes including puberty, male and female menopause, and thyroid conditions. These issues may be creating circumstances that make it difficult to function at the usual pace. These cycles occur to both men and women at different phases in life. Teens going through hormonal imbalance may develop the symptoms and experiences listed. The parents, guardians, and society working with teens may notice that there is a lack of working synapses.

The aging-brain population presents challenges as the process occurs. Being able to determine the difference between tenacity and belligerence will be up to the family, friends, and others. It is nearly impossible to advise those who insist they have lived through it all and know everything. It can be especially difficult when the decision affects their perceived freedoms, like giving up driving. Acting appropriately in the present diverse society may not be simple for someone who has grown up in a different time and world. Aging brain cells may not function as quickly or efficiently.

Times have changed and there are differences between the past and the present. Recognizing these changes can be nearly impossible for the person with an aging brain. Living in long-term memory becomes evident to others. When someone is limited to conversations that are rooted in the past with only glimpses of the present and little notice of the future, the reliance on long-term memory becomes evident.

Brain Tired

"Brain tired, brain exhausted, or brain cluttered" are not yet medical diagnoses. Research in this area has only recently begun. There is a rapidly growing population suffering from the initial symptoms, which include poor judgment, exhaustion, and slow and reduced decision-making ability. STRESS is a major cause. Stress changes the brain's ability to function and filter the information stream. Behavior is altered by the biology and chemical balance in the brain.

People who are brain tired have too many balls in the air; too many hours on electronic devices; too many stressful moments during the days, weeks, and months. The exhausted person sees no end in sight. So play the airplane game: lighten the load, reduce the calendar of events, and turn off the power to the electronic devices. Sit back and rest until a new elevation is reached. The habit of being expected to constantly add to your plate has become the normal situation. This pattern needs to be broken. Finding a balance between "busy" and "overload" is elusive but possible.

Do You Know Someone?

Do you know anyone who is experiencing any of these issues? The group who knows anyone or interacts with people in any category is rapidly growing as the numbers in the other categories increase. There will be very few people who never interact with someone in the other three categories. For those who join the group in this last category, the basic requirement is patience.

You may find yourself in the other categories in the future.

Denial is a pleasant thought, though not always beneficial.

What Is Happening?

In a brain like mine, there are smoking circuits, frazzled lines, and connections which are frayed and torn. Then there are layers upon layers of... *IT*... whatever *IT* is in your life. *IT* involves putting on the illusion needed for your lifestyle. Oh wait, *IT* is only a façade. It is only your *IT*. Where is your breaking point? The next millimeter of torque, gram of pressure, or personal moment of trauma applied to the delicate system, and the house of cards will collapse at the speed of light. What slight change will destroy the delicate balance?

Now is the time to assess.

Take a moment, grieve briefly, for who you were--and then turn to revel in who you are now. Move forward. Forward is in front of you.

We all get something special to deal with in this lifetime. No one gets through unscathed. The choices are found in how we deal with life experiences.

Effects and experiences of each brain injury or period of brain exhaustion are individual, day-by-day, moment-by-moment, circumstance-by-circumstance. The damage, the location, each unique brain and the relationship to the environmental demands, affect the outcome. Learning to train your brain to use new patterns in daily life is also an individual and personal experience. If nothing is done, nothing changes.

Just when you think you have a handle on something and life is progressing smoothly... some moment arises and your system is challenged. As any day progresses, at any moment, with any circumstance, a system failure may occur.

System failure can be recognized by the blank look, the long pause, or an incoherent phrase that is probably best not to repeat.

Fear sets in. Denial is the next phase. What happens if . . . ? Who will be there for me? How do I recognize the changes? How will I support myself? Why me? Not me . . .

Fear, Anger, Frustration

Yes, these are possible, at any moment and to any extent. Your life has changed. You are not the same, your reactions are not the same, your abilities may have changed and you may never be the former you again. With this realization, the acceptance of the truth will help you to maintain balance and function when dealing with fear, anger and frustration. Ask yourself these things: How far into these places do you want to travel? How long do you want to stay immersed in the emotions? How long does it take to get back to neutral? How does your brain deal with the new stresses? What boundaries have changed?

Ranges of emotions from joy and love which can escalate into anger and even violence have variables based on the locations and amount of damage in the brain. The results can be wildly different.

An emotional swing that is uncommon would be an important time for assessment. Assess yourself, work with trusted family and friends, and when appropriate seek professional assistance. Consider all available options and try strategies until you discover what works best for you. Each situation will require an assessment and the creation of strategies.

Maybe there is a need for a new outlet to challenge your brain. Try something new. Sometimes taking a rock-climbing course, learning to mountain bike, participating in a salsa class, or taking drumming instruction or horse-riding lessons will drastically change your outlook on the world.

Create times to release anger and frustration to make the emotions more manageable. It takes time to unwind from frustration and anger. By building endurance and tolerance as you develop strategies, it is easier to solve issues before they escalate.

When a full emotional moment occurs, the stress levels in the brain increase.

When my daughters were young, we had an understanding in the family. Anger and frustration were acceptable emotions. However, they were to be expressed in the comfort and privacy of their bedroom. If they were in public, they were to wait for the appropriate location and time to "pitch a fit."

If they wanted to debate on an issue, anger and frustration levels needed to be assessed continually. If necessary, they were expected to leave the situation, then wait patiently until there was a reduction of emotional overwhelm, organize their thoughts, and return to the situation.

Learn to control yourself. Learn to leave. Learn to back away. Learn to calm your brain. Lean to reset your brain.

When you start to hit the emotional wall, assess. Assess yourself, your environment, your strategy to be safe, secure and supported. You will need to practice.

Where to Start

Stop, breathe and assess! Give your brain time to respond. Thinking you can step on the gas pedal and fly down the autobahn of life in your Ferrari may not be as possible as it once was and certainly probably not as safe. Breakdowns are bound to happen. Don't be afraid to pull over to the side of the road for a moment. Proceed slowly to prevent frustration.

Frustration indicates you are attempting to rush your brain processes and it is not working well. Step away when emotions or physical responses start to reach uncomfortable levels. You can always come back and return to the task. Give yourself time to reset the system and start again. This can occur in a matter of seconds. However, resetting is a skill that has to be learned, organized and practiced.

Brain overload is a personal thing and can happen in a moment which can limit your ability to control yourself and your environment. It happens when there is too much of anything or everything going on. It can vary and act without rhyme or reason and become uncontrollable. Overload may be embarrassing or inconvenient for you and the people around you.

It is what it is. It is not the end of the world.

In the middle of the tornado, find compassion, gratitude, and laughter. Your group of family and friends will learn that you are okay with your mistakes, foibles, and "oopsies." Mistakes are acceptable and unavoidable. They are part of the process. Your family and friends will teach others, and eventually the whole world will know that we all have these moments and it is okay.

I personally find that letting myself have a panic attack and hyperventilating into a cold sweat is time consuming and makes the whole situation worse. The recovery time is huge.

Laughter assists in many circumstances to remove the edge and shift the gears in the brain. It takes a level of relaxation to laugh. What is the alternative? The decision of how to respond is a choice. Choose your battles.

You don't realize what you don't know until you are faced with a task which requires a compromised skill or missing bit of necessary knowledge. Suddenly you draw a blank spot and you find yourself in a mental hole. It is as though you are expected to climb a mountain in winter and you are wearing Bermuda shorts.

Create strategies to climb out of the mental hole and complete the tasks to which you are assigned. Developing a variety of skills will help in daily life over the coming years. Acknowledge that not everything will be finished on time, do what you are able to complete today, and learn to communicate with others for help. Tomorrow will offer time for you to work on something else that needs your attention.

Determination, tenacity, endurance, compassion, and gratitude are crucial to the ability to function and participate fully in daily life.

Taking control in your life involves change. Accepting the change is the total responsibility of the individual and the process is learned, organized and practiced. It will be a continual, repeated process to learn or relearn a single task.

I have had to relearn how to use my tape recorder every time I pick it up. I have to read the instructions again and again. I have yet to be able to listen to anything stored on the recorder because I don't remember how. Someday I will take time to learn that skill. These skills are constantly being challenged with the new electronic devices appearing in my life.

I think, WOW, I am learning something new all the time!

I live in the here and now. I know that is all there really is.

Education, re-education, and continuing education are necessary. Have patience, one day at a time. It is all anyone has.

Moment of Awareness

(Please take this page and make notes as needed)

Memories

Memories are those precious strings that tie us close to the people and experiences in our lives. These strings can be unexpectedly frayed or cut at any single moment of time.

I like to think that memories lost allow room for new memories, which I forget later.

Don't be afraid to admit that you do not remember.

I have to admit my short-term memory loss many times every day. It takes me a long time and many meetings to remember a name and that memory may last only for a short time. New memories may slip away. New thoughts may be fleeting. The events that occur in a day may be gone by nightfall. Waking each day begins a new page of thoughts that may disappear into thin air or stay with me for a time. It helps to establish, repeat and use these new patterns throughout the day. These patterns allow me to organize sequences of movements and use them repetitively to live as independently as possible.

When I leave the driveway, my car goes to the office. There are times when I am not going to work and still find myself in my office parking lot.

I say you do not need to clog up the brain with a bunch of old memories. Leave room for the here and now to be present.

Live with awareness of your surroundings and pay attention to the task you are performing.

When you want to remember and can't, it is frustrating. Stress seems to reduce skill levels. Stop and assess; give yourself a few moments. Let it all go. The more pressure you place on yourself to recall or to think, the more you experience the vacuum and the sense of loss. Breathing and giving yourself time will help to put the pieces together.

Some of the last memories to slip away as you age are music and your name.

Buy and wear kneepads; there may be times when you will be praying. These may help.

I taught a class once and by the end of the two days, I was calling everyone in the class "Lisa." It was the only name I remembered. There was no one named Lisa in the class.

Attention Span

What?

Focus; what a nice thought. When learning to focus, you might have an attention span that lasts seconds, minutes, or hours. When the distractions are minimal and the subject is interesting, your attention span will be longer. When your focus is waning, add something new to the topic, try a new plan of action, or take a short break. Keep working through the chores until they are completed, taking breaks as needed. Mix up your favorite chores with the one you like least or is most difficult. The things you need the most are usually more difficult and produce a slight elevation in stress. Slow the process down and take a short rest break as needed.

Continuing to push through the task when your concentration is broken will likely produce little more than a blank stare or frustration. This holds true for both sides of the situation, you and the others who are present. You may be able to accomplish more with greater ease and accuracy if you take short breaks and enlist assistance from someone as needed. Begin to recognize when it is appropriate to ask for help. Choose your need for assistance with care and caution.

Moment of Awareness

(Please take this page and make notes as needed)

Family, Friends, and Others

Dear Family and Friends,
There is nothing we would love more than to be as capable as we once were. We are scared and need your support through the changes we are experiencing.
Love, Us.

We all need to take time to find compassion for those who are watching the changes and those who have to live inside this new world. Learning to understand the path of others is an art. This path may be confusing for those who engage in activities and share lives with people having brain issues.

Monitor as the circumstances change. We want to maintain as much of our lives as possible.

Everyone is learning at the same time.

Find resources you can trust.

For family and friends, watching the process of our learning as it occurs may include seeing frustration, hopelessness, and whining. It is okay. There is a fine line between helping and taking over the whole task.

Providing too much outside assistance may limit the person's internal process of learning. Remember learning simple tasks in elementary school? Remember learning to write cursive? Who held the big pencil? It may take time and practice to master the new skills. Beneficial outcomes require communication with the brain and then allowing time for the brain to respond. Each person has a different response time for each incident. Wait a few moments to observe whether the need was taken care of, before assisting. This is not always an easy task. Yes, you could have it done in a matter of seconds. We need to do it ourselves anyway.

Your help may be required. We, the brain issues group members, have to keep challenging ourselves, or the losses domino.

This delicate matter requires your observation and communication.

Family, friends and people with brain issues,
Help!
Ask for help!
Accept help!
Participate in the help!

Friends and family, don't assume anything. There may be changes in the level of function at **any** given time. Begin to recognize the moments when circumstances start to rise and how the brain issue group member is not capable of dealing with them. Use this opportunity to advance your observation skills and communication.

Assessment of each individual situation is necessary.

Find the teaching style that is most successful and comfortable for you and use it. When communicating information either by visual, audio or tactile means, put as much information into the appropriate format as possible. Make learning as simple and stress free as possible.

The perception I have of my world and I have of your world, and the perception you have of my world, are occurring through our own filters. Some changes may be subtle for the observer but monumental to the observed. If I go out of the house leaving a verbal list of chores for my teenage daughter, nothing will get done. If I leave a written list on the refrigerator the chores are completed and checked off. Assessment and communication within her learning style alleviated some stress in her ability to process information.

Remember, **because you can**, that we have gaps which need bridges. We would like to have a total picture. We put the pieces we have together and may think we have a total picture. What you want is not always relevant to what is possible. We do not process information in the same way we used to, or even as you think we will based on what we have done in the past. You have to change your expectations. There may be no regularity or consistency in the new course of action being planned and taken. Suggestions may not be welcomed and may even be taken as impositions.

Have patience and compassion. We are doing what we are able to do and may think we are doing everything perfectly.

Sometimes everything is a hit for months and then we totally miss.

Take time to assess.

Is this information helping?

Caretaker Burnout

Everyone will, at some point in their lives, encounter people with brain issues requiring assistance from caretakers. Caretakers come in all ages, sizes, races, and backgrounds. Family members, neighbors, and friends are usually the first layer of help. When the needs become greater than the time and energy of this layer, professional help or assisted living becomes necessary.

As a person with experience working with someone with brain issues. I can attest that caretaker burnout becomes an enormous ongoing issue.

Expectations that brain issue group members need to be waited on hand and foot all of the time is false, most of the time. Take time to make pleasant moments.

Brain issue group members, take strides to do as much as possible for yourself. Movement is necessary to keep one's brain working efficiently. Caretakers assist in the forward movements of people who would prefer to stop and mentally deteriorate.

Caretakers are expected to be kind, compassionate, giving people. Sometimes by giving too much they compromise themselves, to the point of exhaustion.

Be generous with your caretakers.

Use kind words, gratitude and compassion to thank caretakers for the opportunities they create for you. With their help, the outside world becomes a safer and more accessible, more comfortable place for everyone.

Acknowledge when they are correct. Arguing is exhausting for everyone.

Make a decision to commit to a comfortable level of independence in which both your and your caretaker's lives are functional and simple. Establish lines of communication and make action plans that create win-win situations for everyone.

Take time apart from each other to participate in activities which bring pleasure and relaxation. Time apart will help you to remember how much appreciation you have for each other and to return with stimulating new conversations.

As a caretaker, if you live in or work for extended time frames, burnout is common.

Attend to your own physical and mental health first. Take time off before you reach the end of your rope. Know your limitations and boundaries. Designate free time throughout the day and make space for your personal life.

Find responsible substitutes to allow time away when necessary so you are able to participate in your own activities and feel stress free when gone.

Everyone needs to shoulder his or her own responsibility as much as possible.

Responsibility assists everyone during the process of maintaining self-esteem and independence. We all want to be valued and active in our lives.

Unpaid caretakers are a blessing for every minute they spend and everything they do for someone else. They have made a decision to fill their precious time with assisting you. This means they are unable to do something for themselves or someone else during this time. Say thank you frequently.

Paid caretakers are qualified individuals with specific job tasks and assignments. They get a paycheck. Take time to understand the relationship and the expectations of the job description. Along with their check should be your gratitude and smiles.

In both cases the caretaker has certain tasks to perform. This does not include indulging your every whim and following your every order. Consider the caretaker's limitations and capabilities. Think carefully about what is necessary and about what is optional. Assess your needs and capabilities along with the caretaker's skills to make a functional list of tasks.

Do all that you are capable of doing. Be tenacious and allow the caretaker to assist when needed. Self-sufficiency is a fantastic and rewarding experience.

Make a commitment to your life. Be honest with yourself. Do you want a caretaker or crutch?

Moment of Awareness

(Please take this page and make notes as needed)

Observations

Regular assessment needs to occur on an ongoing basis.

There will be changes that make no sense to those observing. Some newfound sensitivities and differences in the way a person with brain issues experiences the environment may become more obvious than others.

A brain issue group member may experience a new hypersensitivity to seemingly random stimuli. For example, awareness of fabric in contact with the skin, certain colors, patterns, or textures may invoke stress on some level.

There are moments when I am standing in my room with the contents of my closet dumped on the bed and the floor. I am struggling to choose an outfit for the day. I have tried on everything and nothing feels right. It is time to leave for a gala event and I am standing in my favorite jeans and comfy sweater because that is all I am comfortable wearing.

Touch may be difficult. You may be sensitive. There are many forms of massage, bodywork, physical therapies and somatic practices using varied levels and amounts of touch. Physical contact may assist in the development of self-awareness. Too much physical contact may overstimulate and reduce the effectiveness of the touch. The fine line between the two is subjective. Work that has more specific contact and neurological connection for the client may assist in the development of awareness and change.

Being in a room with too many people talking may be overwhelming. Background music, television or street noise can overload the auditory system. Though someone is attempting to speak with me, I have no idea what that person is saying. Good luck. Find a quiet space for important conversations in order to be able to focus on the topic.

Spatial concepts may change. It may become difficult to navigate through space with ease. Walking in a hallway with patterned carpet, wallpaper, and fluorescent lighting may overload and overwhelm.

To combat this, try touching the wall as you walk, running a finger down the wall for ease in balance. Focus your eyes on something and reduce the picture to a manageable size.

Ask yourself and those you care for the questions necessary to assess if information has been received. Then realize there is a distinct possibility the information is only partially retained and maybe even only for a fleeting moment. Be prepared to patiently repeat, and repeat and repeat your comments. This is an important concept. Think of it as an exercise in patience. Do not worry, sometimes we forgot we answered the question and won't get upset with your prying.

When you are fully engaged in an activity there is an intense presence of focus at work. You may observe this intensity when you are learning and relearning something. Your tenacity may be loud.

Because it was okay yesterday does not mean it is okay today.

At times you may wonder why we haven't taken care of a specific task. We are not able to.

If the task is reduced to smaller steps or chunks we may be able to accomplish the task. Again . . . that would be *maybe*.

Realize there is a hole in our system that does not allow the sum of all the parts to equal the expected total any longer.

Mail delivery happens daily. Each day in comes a pile of letters, advertisements, catalogues, magazines, and junk mail. Most bills include marketing information for something along with the billing statement. A brain issue group member may sit and look at the nice pictures, ending up with a pile of paper on the table or the counter or next to the chair then moving it to a box. The statements eventually will end up in the pile of advertisements in the recycling. The bill becomes delinquent and late fees and charges are applied because there is too much stuff in the envelope that is distracting.

Take a second look at the situation. We are not able to complete all the tasks we used to do any longer.

This is a delicate situation.

It may take time to realize how large the hole is or how it relates to tasks of the past. Have patience with us.

In conversation, it helps to have as many cues as possible, including being able to look at the face, read the lips, and include as much of the body language as possible. Telephones are more difficult to hear and integrate what is heard. Modifying the pace and tone of language may help to facilitate communication.

My father could not hear high tones and my mother could not hear low tones. They could not hear each other unless they were looking at each other. They eventually realized they had to make changes in their voices based on non-verbal communication cues. Yelling from another room does not mean anyone heard your conversation.

I can hear better in my left ear, but I have a harder time processing what is said. I can process what is said in the right ear, but I don't hear as well. Go figure. Sound-canceling stereo headphones are fantastic. WOW, I actually hear a movie or music.

Reading may become difficult. The brain and the eyes may not be functioning as well together. Font size, color of writing, color of paper, and illustrations make reading easy or impossible. Looking at a page of letters and numbers in beige ink on light green paper may appear as a blur or may not be visible to the person with brain issues. It is difficult to process and integrate the words on the page. Black on white may be easier for many of us. Contrast is good.

I was sitting with a group of people in a restaurant and the menu was written in red script print on a white page. The majority struggled to distinguish the words on the page. Fortunately there were a few who translated the menu for the rest. Text and paper colors can affect those without brain issues as well.

Some of the reading circuits may not work as well. Start reading materials at a level which makes reading easy and pleasurable. It may be the primary school books with one word on each page. Learn to read again. Be tenacious. Start all over again. What else do you have to do with your spare time? Some brain issue group members are able to use flash cards or play letter games when riding in the car; others are not. Find a way to make the impossible possible. Take time to find ways to meet your personal needs and abilities. Be patient, be kind.

Learn the letters, learn the sounds, make the sounds, and combine the letters into words. Keep going. It takes time to read the words and formulate the sounds in the brain. It is yet another process to make them with the tongue and mouth.

In 2003, as part of my brain injury, my diagnosis included Pseudo Foreign Accent Syndrome. At that time, I had 52% intelligibility, meaning that half of the time my speech was understandable. It has been a long road to learn to speak again. When I am tired, my speech patterns are difficult to understand and my accent becomes more prevalent.

When I am tired, my vision alters and one eye seems to float without clarity. I have been through periods where I had double vision. Driving is dangerous with double vision, so I had to stop driving and have someone drive me. It is best to err to the side of caution. Avoid creating havoc when help is available.

Rest is the answer, the only answer when one becomes overwhelmed.

Brilliant minds make rehabilitation tools, brain tests and games for brain-injured people. Some of the things they create need to have minor adjustments to make them simpler and more effective. The creators do not always understand the intricate and delicate differences necessary to make learning possible on a daily basis. Many people do not have the ability to articulate their needs.

Brain injured, brain tired or brain fogged does not mean there is a lack of intelligence. It means it takes longer to activate, integrate, and communicate.

Some of the areas of the brain may become more functional to make up for the deficit. Again, it might not happen completely. Each situation becomes a day-to-day, moment-to-moment, and circumstance-to-circumstance process. Experience gratitude; it is what it is. It could be worse. There are options.

I am grateful I only sustained the level of damage that I did. With brain trauma, a second more without oxygen, a gram more pressure of impact, a millimeter of difference in location and the damage can be changed profoundly.

I am able to function at the level that I do. With tenacity, I am able to lead a productive professional life, have recently completed a Master's degree, take salsa dancing lessons, participate with my family and friends in a wide variety of activities, travel alone, live alone, spend time alone. These are huge accomplishments in my opinion. I am blessed to have people who surround me and love me. It is all good when you get to the bottom line.

Every single day is the life you have now.

Hearing

I can't hear you...

My freedom depends on my independence. Brain function for the use of all my senses, vision, hearing, taste, touch and smell reduces when there are issues. We are all dependent on the ability for brain function so we can live with ease. As one of the senses diminishes, there is hope the others make up the difference.

Assessments are necessary to evaluate the baseline to know where you are so you have the opportunity to make adjustments and changes. It is easier to change when we know where we are and where we would like to be. Hearing is imperative to our ability to function in the environment. Get a baseline hearing test. There are free testing sites. There are no viable excuses.

My curiosity led me to take the test and discover my ability to hear or not. Hearing is a broad range of information processed by the brain. At the time, my hearing captured a reasonable range of tones and sounds. It was about four years later at Christmas when my daughters suggested a follow up hearing test. "Is it that bad?" "Yes".

It was in the follow up test that I discovered my hearing had deteriorated only a few percentages. The changes were loss in pitch ranges. The pitch ranges included those of my daughter's voices, which might have mattered less if they were teenagers and I didn't want to hear.

My hearing was adequate but I struggled. Listening to the phone, eating in a restaurant, attending a gathering, going to a concert, watching a movie, and focusing on conversation were becoming more difficult. My aging mother has hearing aids and chooses not to wear them as them make her 'look old." Would I succumb to the embarrassment of aging, being deaf and pretending all is well?

I started wearing glasses when I needed them to see. I change my diet to add more spice as my taste diminishes. My touch and sense of smell slowly must be shrinking at a pace that is below notice. Why do I have such a hesitation to augment my hearing? Vanity? Insanity?

Most importantly, what I was missing flooded my thoughts. Silence slips slowly into our life, without notice, fading your ability to notice the sound refinement and depth away until there is silence. Hearing loss is largely due to brain function that does not happen any longer. It is not just damage to the inner ear, middle ear or drums. It is the brain not being able to hear and process sound and language.

Why struggle? Why work so hard in an attempt to understand the conversation? When you in a crowd, are you able to hear the person who is speaking to you? Can you hear the delicacy of music? The birds singing? Are you safe when walking down the street? What are you missing?

Next, my curiosity wandered to the effect of my hearing or lack of it held on my balance. Prior to my hearing aid fitting appointment, I filmed myself walking forward, backwards, with my eyes open and closed. I walked on a parking curb in the same patterns. I also filmed the mobility and flexibility in my neck and upper body. There is a small rotation in the neck and upper body in order to turn the good ear closer to maximize the ability to hear. This rotation may be one of the causes of unexplained chronic pain in the neck.

How will the little hearing buds assist in balance? Yes. There was a remarkable difference in the neck mobility and flexibility. Walking was far more stable without the falling side to side and leaning when in gait.

It was a bit of a shock to find that having the two little hearing pieces in my ears improved my ability to walk with clear and concise steps forward with more ease. Fear of falling reduces because I am not falling off balance as often when I walk.

Being able to attend meetings, work with clients, hear the dialogue on the phone and hear my own speech. This will continue to assist me in improvement of my speech patterns and reduce my stress when in a group or challenging situation.

I suggest a baseline-hearing test for everyone. Once you know where you are, you will be able to plan. Hearing is a huge portion of brain health.

Rest

Rest is one hope for change in the brain.

Rest is an internal state of calm, not a place in the external world. This place is the moment where you are able to breathe and sink into a status of quiet. There is a lack of tension in the body, a place of tranquility when everything just quietly works and you are at ease.

It is during the times of rest that the brain has time to review and integrate the information received. Continued pushing through the schedule and lists adds more and more information without processing of the current information.

The challenge is to find time to rest. Overwhelm happens during the constant information blasting on your senses and bombarding both the subconscious and conscious minds. Taking the time to rest is a great challenge when the preference is to push through the barriers and continue to persevere.

It awakens the two-year-old in all of us when we remember the infamous "nap-time" option for an afternoon.

Rest may be simply stopping to take a full breath, preferably three. There will be times when you need to lay down and take a nap.

We need time to allow the brain to catch up to the action. Attempting to bypass this important moment may lead to feelings of being overwhelmed and frustrated.

When I began to ride horses, the first time I rode was for one hour. On the twelve-mile drive home, I considered stopping on the side of the road and sleeping. As soon as I got home, I made it to the bed and slept for eight to ten hours. My brain was exhausted from all of the subtle balancing required to stay on the horse. There is enormous brain activity involved in the integration of a completely new endeavor.

Rest is a learned activity. Learn to take time for nothingness.

Create a routine for going to bed and sleeping. Make the bedroom a place to sleep. Ensure the space is quiet enough to rest. Remove the television, phone, and computer screens; instead put up beautiful pictures. Make the room dark and reduce the sound.

Some people need "white noise" to sleep. There are many forms of white noise; some may be more restful than others. Going to bed is different from going into the bedroom to watch television or work on the computer. Reduce the number of electronic devices in the bedroom.

Parents provide a routine for their child's bedtime. It is okay to continue to develop a bedtime routine appropriate for adults. Sleeping may need to be learned and planned.

Take care of the difficult tasks when rested and when the brain is functioning at its peak.

Sleep

Sleep is the best and may be the only time for the body and brain heal. Interrupted sleep patterns, restless sleep, not dropping into the deep rest state reduces the healing and functional ability of the brain. Pain is one of the factors that keeps us from comfortable deep sleep.

Evaluate your bed, bed linens, and bedroom environment. Is this restful and peaceful. Consider the support necessary to optimize your rest and wellbeing. Change your mattress if it has seen better days and increases your discomfort.

Choose bed linens with consideration to fabric content and fibers, weight, and coziness. Some people require more weight covering them while they sleep. Clean your linens regularly to keep this area of your home fresh and ready to receive your exhaustion and need for quiet rest.

Asses the functional use of the adjustable base bed in your life.
The transition from sitting to lying and back up to sitting is extremely difficult for many. The need to make this transition often all night long creates more pain and stress. Having options for the height of your head and feet with more support than a pile of pillows. Less effort and stress.

If you are needing Caretaker support, the adjustable base is a tool for them as they assist in moving people from standing to sitting to lying and up again. They are not old-style hospital beds.

New modern adjustable beds are elegant support systems for comfortable living into your future.

Sleeping environments require reduced light, electronics and sound. Some need to have white noise to rest. Attempting to rest with the television news blaring is difficult. Take the big black eye out of the bedroom or cover it with something when sleeping. Replace the television with something soothing to observe when drifting off to sleep or waking.

Sleep for hours, this may necessitate going to bed earlier as there may be fewer variables demanded by the waking hour. Prior to bed, take a shower to wash away the outer world. When you lie down, begin slow movements and breathing to release the tension and influences and events from the day. Make a pleasant quiet down routine that separates the day and beginning of the rest period. This is not a natural occurrence, it is learned and practiced.

Making these changes in my daily life created more BrainEase during my waking hours. My productivity and ability to function in many environments improved noticeably.

Honor yourself, create your incredible sleep world to heal.

Activities

There is a need to participate in activities. You need to be active. Movement is imperative to activate brain cells. It may be a change from the sedentary lifestyle. What is difficult may be what benefits you most. To be honest, when it is difficult, who wants to move? It is so easy to sit and fade into the deep places of your brain forever.

There is also the tendency to make excuses about why exercise or movement is not happening. Too tired, too much to do, too sore, too overwhelmed, too stressed, too . . . too . . . too . . .

Honestly, it may be that participating will require time, ability and understanding of the expectations of the activity. Initially being involved in activities may be too much to think about. Learning a new activity might demonstrate the new difficulties one has when competing with others. We are trained to want to be the first place winner. Potentially, failing is a terrifying possibility.

By changing your perspective on what constitutes a success, each step in creating a healing lifestyle can be seen as progress. Perhaps it would be helpful to look at your ability to learn individual steps of an activity. As the components are learned, combining them together in a new pattern will help build success. For example, remembering the steps in a foxtrot is the goal. Figuring out which foot is left and which is right may be first in the process toward the goal. Be kind, gentle and patient with yourself as the process happens. Two steps forward and one step back is common. These steps forward and back become the dance.

Activities come in many forms. There are activities that are incorporated into your daily life. These may change when your brain function is altered. Find an activity about which you have passion. Take a moment or two each day and focus on one aspect of the activity. Find something that is difficult, preferably not impossible. Begin with a step that is comfortable and start practicing.

Shake it up!

When you walk, try using walking sticks. Not as though they were canes to lean on but to assist you with balance and support. You make walking easier. Think "left" with every left foot stride. Think "right" with every right foot stride.

Read out loud. Children's books are fantastic at providing foundation by starting with easier words. Dance alone, dance with a partner, dance an organized step or just tap a toe or finger in rhythm with the music. Try a new sport; ride a horse; take a Feldenkrais, Bones For Life, or yoga class. Stir with the opposite hand. Touch different surfaces and focus on the individual qualities of these surfaces. Learn to knit, crochet, tie flies, paint, use a new program on the computer, find a constellation, count birds, or train a dog to do a new task. You will notice when you regularly make a list of activities, the possibilities are endless.

Find a way to live that allows you a little spare time to pursue something new. It doesn't mean you need to knit everyone you know a sweater. Start with a single stitch. The actions required to cast the yarn on the needle, loop other yarn around your finger, and move the needles in an organized manner will be enough.

Leave it and rest. Come back to it or choose another task. Shake it up. This does not mean that you buy all kinds of new hobbies and supplies. Two chopsticks and a piece of twine will do to learn knitting. The challenge and the learning come from the process of learning to pay attention to the details. It may take weeks before the process integration becomes evident in the response from the body and the brain's memory banks.

Move and act with purpose. Play with these concepts. Play as a child with the curiosity and new eyes for looking, ears for hearing, and hands for touching, experiencing the wonderment of life for the first time. You have worked. People approach play with different attitudes. Hurrying and forcing the issue will reduce the creative juices and the ability to allow you to process the new information.

These are good times for lots of laughter. When the process becomes difficult, the learning begins. You already know the easy stuff. You are capable in those arenas. Now, to build a larger map of pathways, the areas you don't know well will have to be explored. Be kind and gentle with yourself. This may be exhausting, frustrating and challenging. Yahoo, the fun begins!

When the fun is overwhelmed by the difficulty, know that the timing of the activity might be incorrect. Sometimes there is a vital piece of information missing. This piece may have to be found before you can return to the activity with ease.

I am working on Sudoku. When I started, I continually mixed up the numbers 3, 5, 6, 8, and 9. They all looked alike. This time when I picked up the easy book, my focus time was several minutes. It was possible to work on a line or two at a time. Each day a few numbers go on the page. My progress is fantastic.

Count your blessings and appreciate the small differences and changes you are making. One way or another, things will change. It may be more empowering to have some control in what changes are yours.

School

Years are spent in the educational system from preschool through high school and continuing into vocational schools, colleges and universities.

Yes, we assume that all the brain-issue group members are the ancient people who are residing in assisted living homes. Instead, we need to look around at the people in our immediate environment.

Let's begin with our children. There is brain overload happening in all age groups. The number of screens, games, toys, phones, texting, twittering, networking, exams, expectations to perform at high levels, and hormones contribute to overload and create brain chaos.

When they finish the day at school, there may be homework. They may need a protein snack and a short break before completing homework. Which is more brain tiring: a chapter of history and writing a book report or spending several hours playing video games, texting and television?

My younger daughter at about five years old began reading chapter books, going from large print to small print. Her eyesight was not yet developed enough to be able to focus on the smaller print and she was having difficulty reading. An eye exam provided the solution, giving her glasses until her eyes moved from more farsighted to normal vision over the following couple of years. Young children looking at the small electronic device screens may need to have monitoring to avoid damage and exhaustion from eyestrain.

Puberty adds a huge number of people into the brain issue group.

Expectations to live up to the parent's dreams to perform the unbelievable tasks, to be the stars in sports or music or dance, and to obtain education have overtaken the reality. Adolescents are people who need to develop and grow in healthy bodies, minds and spirits.

Where is rest? Where is the space of quiet to relax, think and be creative? When do parents stop the mania and take responsibility to set boundaries for the children who are not old enough to know how?

My daughter came home from university without the ability to sleep. It took two years before she began to develop a more organized sleep pattern. Three years later there are still many nights lacking sleep.

School is a microcosm of the working world. Students learn to stand in line, take what information is present and expand it with the time spent on homework and outside activities. It takes time to build stamina to focus and participate for hours in anticipation of working in the future.

Students are expected to associate with people of different cultures, beliefs, religions, and academic abilities, and to learn tolerance. The learning environment requires students to work with people whom they do not like and many who do not like them. Diversity in cultures, languages, religions, and behaviors are daily factors requiring energy and patience for students. Students in the pre-teen years through early twenties may lack sufficient brain development to logically and maturely interpret situations easily. Time spent in school builds the necessary endurance for expected time spans involved in the daily work world. School prepares people for life; it is not perfect and neither is life.

A student's primary job is school.

Teens are driving their siblings and friends after limited sleep and a night of video games, television, and computers. They may have enjoyed something to eat, an energy drink, their medications, along with a liter of soda. The only thing on their mind is racing hormones, the final exam they did not study for and a party happening this coming weekend. They are brain tired, stressed and overwhelmed before they turn the key of the ignition. They are in the driver's seat of the family auto with passengers all talking, listening to music, texting, and eating. Who is paying attention to the demands of traffic and the road?

To meet the requirements of educational systems it is highly desirable to have the optimal number of brain cells to memorize, categorize and utilize the learning experience to the fullest. Tests and exams are built into the process as an additional venue for developing brain patterns that differ from studying alone or in groups. Life is filled with moments where these skills are utilized. People with brain issues may have difficulty focusing for periods of time, or listening to lectures, or lengthy visual stimulation. Breaks are not always available when the student feels the need to rest. These same issues are present when working.

Activities including sports, gym, and clubs, are prevalent in the personal and social networks for children and teens. Occasionally there are accidents when participating in activities. Head injuries may be an outcome. Shaken brain, multiple head impacts and concussions are common. Assess carefully when an impact occurs. Look for subtle changes in speech, behavior, personality, and balance. Be in contact with a medical professional if there are questions or if changes become obvious in the injured person.

My brother crashed his bike when he was seven years old. He spent a week in the hospital with a concussion. When he got out of the hospital there was never any further mention of the accident and he moved on. When he was about fifty-five years old he asked me if I thought some of his difficulty with school, especially math, might have been from the concussion. Take note of changes after an accident and continue to assess for an extended period.

Assess to determine how many activities a person with brain issues can handle before they reach the tipping point where the brain gets overloaded and they are unable to function effectively. Learn to make difficult choices and experience limits and boundaries. These are hard lessons to learn and they remain constantly relevant.

Going back to school or taking classes as we age is a fantastic way to practice organizing thoughts. Challenge the daily routine and life processes. There are classes in the community colleges, recreation facilities, senior centers and community centers. Choose subjects that interest you. Expand your thoughts and open opportunities for new experiences. You are only limited when you choose to stop growing. Tenacity is one path.

Work

Profession, career, or job, this position is one of the major influences in life. It carries our public image of our self and the ability to produce income to survive. Our education, training and skill are in line to produce years of support and relationship to the world. Social and professional alliances are formed through experiences during the workweek.

What happens when your brain is unable to perform the tasks required? What happens when your fellow employees or boss notices changes in your performance? What happens when you face your own limitations and realizations? What happens when you are unable to work and have to change to earn income to live?

Comparing a school day and an average workday, an adult has built the time endurance to hide the exhaustion more effectively. There are higher stakes in the adult world with the responsibility for families, expenses, and mortgages all looming overhead each day. How long can you hide your difficulties? What happens when you live in denial that you have changed?

Routines are important for maintaining balance in the daily schedule. It is much easier to live within an organized program of events than it is to start new every day. When the routine is disrupted we are outside our comfort zone. Pressure and competition in the daily work environment makes chaos in the brain.

Doing work and having money are important. Peace in the mind is even more important. Find your passion, educate yourself in this work and create the life that is important to you.

Your time and attention have been "bought" by the employer. The expectation is that you will produce a specific amount of work during each day. When there is a brain deficit, this expectation may prove impossible. Depending on the specific brain injury, many people are forced to retire early or downsize their time on the job; the end result is disability and aid of some kind. There may be the need to learn a new path or skill which meets your ability and goals. Changing life skills is common; assess yourself, and make changes.

When the work situation changes or ends, there are many aspects of life to be considered. Schedule and routines are disrupted. Additional burdens are placed on your plate which was already overwhelming. Face the reality of changes to you, your personal image and financial comfort. Financial difficulties are compounded by the increase in the cost of healthcare and insurance.

This is a terrifying time. It is the last place we expect to be.

I was working ten days after my brain injury occurred. Work brought focus to my brain. There was routine, stability, and personal rehabilitation.

Each day of work increased my ability to function in daily life with my family, friends and others. I continue to work. Each day continues to offer opportunities to meet the new challenges and make decisions and choices which will affect my life and those who surround me.

Retirement

Retirement is when you stop working and begin to live a different life.

Are you prepared?

This is a time when change occurs in the routine. Be aware of this lack of repetition. It is easy to become complacent. We sometimes forget to continue growing and developing new thoughts, creating ideas, and working on present and future lifestyle plans.

There is huge emphasis on financial planning for the retirement years, putting money away to support your lifestyle and hopefully to participate in activities. But what is your plan to maintain your brain?

Putting together a brain plan is also imperative. Spend as much time planning your time as you spend planning your finances. Creating a friendship circle, a schedule of activities, and a list of hobbies happens over many years.

If your plan is to retire and take a cruise, you will find there is a shortage of activities for the remaining many years of life. Most of our friends come from working relationships, which quickly fade when we are no longer in daily contact. People are busy with their daily lives and you are away from their routine. They now have to make special time for meeting with you.

Many people retire and plan to travel. An occasional trip to see the relatives or a cruise will be more reasonable than leaving on extended safaris.

The hobbies and activities you participate in during your working life will be the ones you continue to enjoy after retirement. Including a pet for companionship and potential increase in exercise may be a consideration at this time in life.

Time to assess.

If your pre-retirement activity list is only work and home, then home will be the only thing on your list. It takes planning and action to make and complete a bucket list. This is easier if you have a partner. If you are alone, the creation and follow-through may be more difficult, but if you don't do it, the end result will be that you feel lonely.

During your working life, if you fill your calendar with volunteer projects, hobbies, religious activities, or other ways to spend your time, you will have made the retirement pathway easier. These will flow into the hours filled by employment.

Similarly, when a spouse dies, the other has to continue. My father died after 58 years of marriage to my mother. She was alone, but was already involved in her carefully chosen volunteer projects, church, and family which continued to grow and flourish. She travels, participates, and checks things off her bucket list daily. The people surrounding her are always admiring her tenacity and functionality.

Look at your life. What do you see in your personal activity account? How much are you investing in the brain fund? Do you have friends outside of work? Do you fill your calendar with new activities to challenge your brain? Are you assuming that when you retire the world will come knocking at your door to entice you into joining? What is on your bucket list? How often do you update the list? When did you start the list?

It is easy to retire, take the cruise, come home, turn on the television and stay in the chair. It is scary to leave.

It takes organization and planning to fill all the hours in the days, weeks, months and years to come. Many quit in a short time.

Plan your brain fund. Make an ongoing list of life activities. Stretch and do things that challenge you. Dance, sing, learn a language, rock climb, be in nature, visit a foreign country, etc. Your overall brain and physical health will thank you. Driving

Driving is freedom.

Yes, people with brain issues are driving, on the roads and highways and in the parking lots. Does this scare you? It should.

Assess. It is more than your independence. People's lives are at stake. Have honest people ride with you. At the end of the ride, if they jump out of the car hyperventilating, take a hint. You may need assistance.

It may be advisable to have a professional driving assessment by rehabilitation personnel. It may be beneficial to participate in a driving safety class after a brain injury and every few years afterwards to assess your skills. It is imperative to be a safe driver. There should be no question whether you are capable of passing a driving exam.

Just because the speedometer goes above eighty does not mean that your brain is capable of responding to the possible circumstances that might occur at that speed. If you cannot accelerate to the recommended speed because you become too nervous, you may need assistance.

Look at your intake of drugs and alcohol and the amount of rest you've had prior to the outing. Have the confidence to suggest another person drive if there is any question about your ability. This is not the time for ego to take over.

There are strips of highway near my office that make me extremely uncomfortable. I have to take the exit, stop, and reorganize my brain in order to continue. I take extreme caution in my planning and it is now common for me to get off the highway prior to these spots and take side roads through town. Safety and comfort are vitally important for me and for the society that has to interact with me.

Listening to music, talking on the phone, conversing with passengers, or texting while driving may be overload for people with brain issues. It is a huge brain drain to drive at least 60 miles per hour with four lanes of rush-hour traffic in each direction.

My mother now needs to watch the face and even lay her hand on the arm of whomever she is communicating with to hear the majority of the conversation. Not so perfect when she is driving.

As my mother ages we discuss when it is that she feels she is safe driving. What weather conditions, time of day, levels of exhaustion? It is a kind conversation where we share her confidences and fears. She continues to drive with awareness and safety.

Taking away the freedom of driving is a major change. Assess carefully and with caution. There are many factors to consider. Public safety becomes the first priority on the list.

Moment of Awareness

(Please take this page and make notes as needed)

Going Shopping

Friends and family who accompany members with brain issues need to remember the environment may be overwhelming. You could be shopping with the "Houdini Shopper." This can be taxing. Take a moment when entering the store to turn the shopper's cell phone to a loud ring you recognize. When you call us, follow the ring and you will find us, eventually. When distracted by something bright and cheerful, we walk away and off we go. Interesting and pretty things are everywhere.

Communication can become difficult when so many wonderful things surround us. Focus is a challenge and yelling at us does not look good to neighboring shoppers, nor does it help us to perform better.

Group members, check the cart to be certain the items on the shopping list are present. You may have added a few extra things, including the model bat-mobile with all the bells and whistles. Who wrote the list and forgot to put it on? You have wanted one for as long as you can remember. People with brain issues may be easily distracted and need to have limitations and clear boundaries for more ease.

Plan the shopping excursions with an understanding that they are complete when the fun meter breaks. If alone, wandering in the same two aisles for over 200 passes means you need to check out or ask for assistance. If you are with a group and you start to wander out of the store into the mall and away, stop. Look around; wait for the group so the others are not lost.

Lists and planning are helpful. To minimize buying all the things you never had as a child on a single trip, use a list. This idea proves effective when used appropriately. Write a list, take the list, remember to get the list out and read the list. Check the list prior to check out then expect to go all the way to the back corner to get the one item you passed repeatedly on the 200 passes of the two aisles. Now the trick is to get back to the front of the store within a specific time-period and not add more than five new VERY important items to the cart.

At the checkout, remembering the pin number is the challenge. Good luck; it is four numbers. I say, shop often so it is engraved in your brain cells. When you first get the card, buy many small items with individual slips so you can practice. Or you can get an old phone with a similar type of number of pad and practice at home. If you have a lapse in use, it may slip away from your fingertips.

Shopping in the same stores becomes the comfortable pattern. Walking into a different store is a chore. The challenge of finding things in a new store, when you know the location in your base stores, can be overwhelming. Large malls with large open spaces, many floors, store upon store, people, smells, loud constant noise, and constant sensory bombardment, may be overwhelming.

In preparation for shopping extravaganzas, understand that when you reach the end of good focus and concentration is limited, there will be exhaustion at the end of the outing. Eating food along the way is helpful to break up the intensity and energize you to continue shopping with new gusto. Upon arriving home, a lemon drop martini is a good way to relax, "for medicinal purposes." These are words of advice for the people shopping with us.

Hide the E-bay password! E-bay is a mall at the end of the fingertips with none of the mall stimuli and bombardment. There is also the unlimited button pushing, the sense of victory, and the love of packages in the mail. Oh wait; there is the bank account and credit card bill. Be aware; online shopping can be dangerous.

Moment of Awareness

(Please take this page and make notes as needed)

Travel

There are many forms and ways of travel; all require some attention to the details of organization and strategy planning to increase the possibility for success. Travel challenges even the most adept.

Make reservations early, including air, hotel, and car. Make copies of all the itineraries and place them in a folder. Do not put the folder in the cabinet out of sight. Instead, put a label on the folder and put it out in the open where you can find it. I use clear letter-size plastic envelopes for travel so I have all the itineraries, boarding passes, and receipts in one place.

Travel light. Remember, you have to carry everything you are taking with you. Do you need to have that much stuff? Assess. Check your luggage to see if you have more than you can lift into the overhead bin or into the trunk. There is not always help to lift, tote and carry. Sherpas are few and far between.

Know the current rules for your mode of travel. Be at the terminal early; it is easier to wait there than in the car stuck in traffic. Reduce all unnecessary stress.

Carry snacks that provide nutritional support during stressful moments. Sugar and caffeine may not be your best friends. There is enormous sensory overload when out of the regular routine. Be kind to yourself.

When you have more things to dig through, pack, unpack, repack and constantly monitor, there is more effort required.

I found multi-colored mesh bags to organize the extra phone cords, sundries, and loose extra items. As repacking occurred the bags helped remind me to include the phone cords in the luggage. Empty bag means look around. I also carry a power strip for the extra plug space.

Find strategies to travel with ease. When I arrive in an unfamiliar city, I use the hotel shuttle, taxi, or hire a car and driver to deliver me to my first destination. I can unload my belongings, rest, and then proceed with a fresh mind. If the flight is long, I may wait until morning to pick up the rental car. When possible, travel with a GPS to avoid reading a map or printed directions when driving in unfamiliar areas.

Check with your insurance companies so you have appropriate travel-related insurance. Assuming you know your coverage in another state or country, in regards to all the fine print on the rental car, medical, and travel cancelation policies, may lead to very stressful and expensive problems. Mistakes in this arena are very expensive and very stressful.

Yelling at the travel professionals does not change that you were ignorant in the first place.

Planning and being aware is the best solution. It may be a more expensive trip to purchase the appropriate insurance and not use it. But what if you do not have the insurance and have to pay for a medical airlift?

Using a black 21" roll-on suitcase may not be your best bet. There are so many of them in the travel world. You don't want to have to check every bag which circles on the baggage carousel. Buy luggage in another color or decorate your bag for ease in detection. Stress-free traveling means you can find your bag when there are other bags nearby. It is amazing how much all the bags look alike. Become familiar with yours or make it stand out so that only you will pick it up.

A car trip does not mean the whole car has to be completely full with the contents of your home. You are leaving home to look at something else. It may be helpful to have some regular items if you have the room. Remember, what you pack, you have to carry. There may be three flights of stairs and a broken elevator.

There are stores everywhere allowing the opportunity to purchase items you may have forgotten. Most hotels have irons, hairdryers and a variety of sundries for purchase or use.

Life requires reality.

Now that all of the planning is done, you are ready to roll out the door . . . How do you get out of the house?

Moment of Awareness

(Please take this page and make notes as needed)

Getting Out of the House

Take a moment to dream, breathe, be.

Distractions usually occur at the time of departure. Being late is stressful. It creates a need to hurry, move quickly, and increase speed without a positive outcome in most cases.

Now you are ready to leave; the process of assessing the lists and making a decision, that all is complete. Departure can happen. Almost.

When you get in the car and notice you have on your slippers, go back and get shoes. Did you remember to grab all the things on the list? Oh, all but one, back to the house. Where is the cell phone? I am going back to the house again. I just spilled coffee all the way down the front of the white shirt, back to the house. This is a typical morning at my house. It is a miracle I make it to any appointment. I have realized that I often leave the house in slippers, so I have a pair of real shoes at the office. I have basic kits including personal items and other cool very necessary stuff in my car, at the office and at home. When I leave home my concern level is reduced knowing I have everything that is important during the day in multiple locations.

Some days are smoother than others. Maybe the organization the prior evening is insufficient and then maybe something stressful happens and all the organization in the world is for naught.

Be satisfied you have most of the necessary things in the car with you when you leave. I am always amazed at the things I haul around and never use. Most of them are in the car or suitcase because I went back for them and was late as a result. I hope I remember the lesson, someday.

When you find yourself walking in circles or to the car and back to the house more than three times, get in the car and drive away.

It is time to just make a stand and leave.

You can pay for shipping the forgotten item later or buy replacements upon arrival.

Travel challenges the brain. From beginning to end there is a constant need for brain work. All of the new environments to step into and the opportunities of seeing, doing and going are fantastic. Allow for time to get lost and disoriented, and nap time to recover. All will make the whole adventure easier.

Many stop traveling or driving because they have gotten lost and were embarrassed to admit the occurrence to anyone. Find a friend to travel with who understands your capabilities and shortcomings. Be honest so they are able to watch out for you and you for them. Take care of your own stuff and when you are able, assist your traveling companion. When traveling is win-win, more people will participate with you. It removes the "wow" in a vacation when time is spent in the police station or hospital looking for the lost.

Crossroads

Every day we come to crossroads which will affect the future we live. Determining the outcome prior to the event is difficult, even with all the variables present. This is where your tenacity takes precedence and your ability to move forward in the face of adversity takes the front seat. Let nothing stand between you and the goal. It may take more time to complete. There may be side trips or backtracking. Commit to the process and move the mountains. Look to the desired outcome and keep all distractions in perspective. There will be those who want to limit your potential to allow you to remain within their comfort zone. Assess if this is truly your best course of action. Is there satisfaction in living in a box?

Consider the cost to you, your brain, your family, friends and others, and the environment when you lose control.

Fear and frustration are commonplace in my daily life. I create strategies to minimize the time and emotional drain potential.

Decisions and Choices

Do you live the diagnosis or do you live?

For me, there was no diagnosis for almost three years after the incident. The upside to this was I continued to live without any idea I was injured. I did not hear my speech with the accent. To me, my voice sounded just like it did before. There were incidents where I thought I communicated my thoughts to someone else. Instead, I had run the conversation in my mind and not actually included anyone else. It was just me talking to myself and to the others in my mind. I was my own audience. Other times, the words out of my mouth did not match the thoughts in my head. The word order or choice of words was incorrect.

Sometimes I knew there were errors and other times, no. Frustration and anxiety for both the speaker and audience are normal reactions to these incidents. This is difficult for family members, friends and others who are in the general vicinity and attempting to understand. Sometimes family members attempt to speak for you.

Learn these phrases: "This is another attempt to communicate, brought to you by my brain," or "I am having another brain moment." It is we who have to laugh first to allow others to be more comfortable with our mistakes. These moments will exist. Find the innate sense of discovery to look forward to the reality.

It did not occur to me I needed to be tested to drive, that I needed assistance, or that my memory banks were disturbed. I look at the world through my brain. Things change constantly. When I couldn't remember something, another task would come to the forefront and the past fleeting questions were gone. Family and friends, this is when your observations are important. Let us know when our focus is wandering. My daughters clap their hands loudly and say, "FOCUS." This process occasionally has to be repeated. When there is need for more than one repeat, noting the environmental stressors is important. Too much is happening and the ability to focus is reduced. Stop, assess and slow the hurricane down.

Ten days after the maxillofacial surgery that resulted in my brain injury, I drove across the state of Washington to a farrier symposium to work with horses and humans for four days. No one explained that I had experienced brain damage during the operation. I am convinced the driving experience re-installed my ability to drive. Working all the sessions with both people and horses confirmed my professional skills.

As a single parent for years, my responsibility to the lives of my children was foremost. If I was in a coma, I would still have to get up and go to work. It was my responsibility. This was not altered with my brain injury.

It may be a choice to stay home living with an infarction, a dead spot in the brain. It might not be an option to get out of it.

My biggest fear is not being able to get out of the darkness or the void and I am stuck forever in the abyss. There are virtual holes in the brain, and through the process of learning it is possible to bypass the pit-holes. Find holes and either fill them in or go around with new neuro-pathways. Know that there will be more holes.

Keep moving; there are 360 degrees in a circle. If something doesn't work, turn 1 degree or 180. Learn to make small steps in many directions to create inroads to various pathways and open many doors. With all the different movement patterns available, knowing there are options is valuable information. Create optional patterns and strategies. Do this regularly with everyday tasks. What else do you have to do with your free time?

If I didn't do things the way I do them now, how would I organize my life to do things differently?

Challenge yourself. Skydiving could be the second item on the list. There is a huge sense of accomplishment at the moment when the decision is made to take on a new challenge. It grows with the completion. The completion is when you have come to a place when the task is finished, or you have reached a place to ask for assistance. Milestones come in all shapes and sizes. Milestones are reached and your life fills with possibilities.

At what point do the challenges outweigh the benefit to continue? Assess this carefully. Growth occurs when challenges are created, met and surpassed. Take a small step until the small step is possible with ease and then add another small step. Every day is a continuum of learning.

Neuro-pathways develop when attention is paid to the change as it occurs.

Doing the crossword puzzle in a similar pattern every day will not develop a new pathway. Start the puzzle from the bottom and work up or from the right side and work to the left, or use your non-dominant hand to write the letters. Rote thought or activities allow only minute changes. Shake it up.

Develop strategies to alter the same task and create a challenge.

As you walk, focus on the left side. Think left, left, left so all the emphasis is on the left side of the body. Walk for several steps and assess the difference in your attention to the left side. Then shift focus to the right side and follow the pattern of thinking.

When the car runs for miles with one tire in the road rut, it is not calm in the car. Getting the tire out of the rut depends on how deep the rut is and how tall the tire is.

This may be time for assistance.

Take on the biggest challenge early in the day when there is maximum clarity and rest. Once that is addressed, everything else is easier.

Do something new every day. Repeat some of what you learned yesterday. Leave something for tomorrow.

Do what you love, do what you dislike, do something. There are times when nothing works. Laugh and rest. Walk away; let in space to view the situation from another perspective. If the timing is correct, start again. You may have to redo the activity as the biggest challenge the next morning or you might forget for several days. If it comes up again, deal with it then.

Appreciate every step; at least there are steps.

Allow yourself to struggle... a little. Know when to stop struggling. There is a balance between challenge and struggle.

No one has it as easy as it seems from an outside perspective.

This arena affects all of those who are in the brain issues group and those who are in the lives of group members. If you had difficulty making decisions before, now will be no different. If you were able to look at the situation and have an instant epiphany, times have changed. There will still be circumstances where your solutions will shock everyone. Another scenario is that you produce a blank stare, long pause and the unintelligible phrase.

Finding your life purpose helps to organize your behavior and allows a greater possibility to live your values. These concepts make the daily routine much easier to live. All becomes more congruent and makes sense to the brain.

Food, Supplements, Alcohol, and Drugs

This is a huge area. Find the experts.

There are professionals who are trained in these fields. Each of the supplement, drug, and food options has many facets and angles to be considered.

Look for and evaluate your allergies, likes, dislikes, environments, cultures and health issues. These are not to be taken lightly. Drugs, supplements, and food contain chemical, biological, and organic substances that when mixed may produce a reaction that works for or against your body and brain. Today, eating a given combination may be fine; tomorrow the combination might not work well. Consult experts. That does not mean ask anyone who is paid to work at a supplement store. Nutritionists, allergists, naturopaths, and appropriate blood work by your physician are helpful places to begin.

Each food or supplement is usually served in combination with other supplements or foods. This may create problems for some people. Diet and food groups may need to be investigated to produce an individualized diet plan which works for you. Finding the winning combination is difficult on a great day.

Supplement options are varied, some may or may not be beneficial. taking supplements is only useful if they are absorbed into your system to provide a benefit. Discuss with a professional the type of supplement, combinations of supplements, the amount to take, and the process involved to break down, digest, and absorb the nutrients. There are multiple forms of delivery systems for supplements. Each has an effect on the absorption rate. Liquid, powder and pills break down in order to be digested into the system. Find the delivery system that works with your body to acquire the maximum benefit from the supplements you need.

Medications need to be monitored by your physician and pharmacist. Use one pharmacy for all of your prescription drugs and build a relationship with the pharmacist. Check with your primary doctor to make an addition to your records when a specialist adds medication. Check with the pharmacist with each new prescription or over-the-counter drug for dangerous interactions and appropriate dosage.

I had an elderly client who discussed her exhaustion and lack of energy. She mentioned her pill intake per day was over twenty-eight pills, all for a variety of different issues. She questioned when she was given a new medication why none were ever removed from her list.

I suggested that she make an appointment with her pharmacist. Take a grocery bag, put all her medications, supplements and whatever else she was taking into the bag. She took all the prescription drugs, vitamins, herbs, supplements, and homeopathic remedies to her appointment. With appropriate analysis of the total picture, the pharmacist realized that the chemical combination was producing an overdose reaction. Her pill intake was reduced and her energy returned.

The pharmacist is knowledgeable in biochemistry and chemistry, capable of reviewing the overall picture and considering the interaction of all the compounds individually and collectively.

Reading the whole label to find the ingredients may produce information. One might find that a single ingredient does not work well for you specifically.

My mother is highly allergic to shellfish. When her hip was sore, her doctor suggested she take chondroitin and glucosamine. After reading the label we realized that this is a product made almost completely from shellfish. She returned to the doctor and asked if they wanted her to take the supplement in their office so she would be at the doctor already when she went into anaphylactic shock.

Food can be a drug. There are hidden items in processed food that can create havoc in the brain and body. There can be an immediate reaction. Aside from allergies there are reactions to caffeine, high fructose corn syrup, sugar, dyes, additives, and preservatives, all of which are present in many foods. Some foods or food combinations destabilize blood sugars. The term "organic" differs depending on which country is providing the product and their standards for organic production.

There are foods that make the body and brain happy and others that create inflammation and irritation. Observation of food reactions can help to determine which foods are more tolerated and digestible for your own physical and mental systems.

Watch the time frame around meal and snack time. When you find that you have lost concentration, function and sense of humor, you might need to eat. Watch your carbohydrate and protein intake at this time.

When my daughter was in second grade, she was having frequent visits to the principal's office. The usual time was shortly after the morning recess. She had burned all the breakfast carbs and her ability to control her mental concentration was depleted. Her metabolism rate was burning through breakfast too quickly, causing her to lose focus and emotional stability in a few hours. After assessing the situation, we arranged for her to eat protein in the mornings during breakfast. She was then able to maintain through the morning until after lunch without the daily conversation with the principal. The protein-heavy meal provided mental stability and a higher level of function. This led to potential for greater personal success throughout the day.

Alcohol is a broad subject. There is the occasional glass of wine or a beer versus the daily bottle of wine and six-pack of beer. Hard liquor has higher alcohol content in a smaller glass. Use caution; protect the public from your inability to function with the extra stress on the brain.

When you add alcohol to the brain of a group member, the outcome may be difficult to predict. Even when working with all of the mental components functioning at full potential it can be difficult. Be kind to yourself. Learn the word "sip." If you are concerned, hold a glass that is a little more than half-full for the whole evening as an easy way to appear to be participating.

Self-medication is similar. There are many choices that alter brain function.

Choose carefully; learn to say no thank you.

Some of the options may harm the nervous system pathways you have left. Some pathways are not restorable or replaceable.

What works for one person may be inappropriate for another.

Read the labels. Be an informed consumer. Advocate for you and your family members. Find the products that assist in balancing the systems to allow a fuller healthier life at the same time.

Memory problems can lead to forgetting to take prescriptions, supplements, vitamins, and drugs in a timely manner or in the correct order. Meals can be inadequate, forgotten or multiplied.

Systems to provide a schedule are important.

This is an extremely important area to observe when dealing with brain issue group members. When there is a deficit that goes undetected for a long period, it can be potentially dangerous.

Being a part of the team of observers to assess circumstances effecting the environment, activities, and health for people with brain issues is difficult. Often those who make infrequent visits may believe everything appears to be normal. The observer may not have enough information. Spend several days together, challenge the limits, and test the routine.

When you are assessing a person with brain issues, observe with as fresh and objective an eye as possible.

Moment of Awareness

(Please take this page and make notes as needed)

Environment

We live our lives in our homes, work at our jobs, and participate in the world around us. We take safety for granted in these places.

But there are silent dangers that lurk in the corners of our environments. There are toxic chemicals in construction materials, cleaning products, and materials that our clothing and furniture are made from. We are surrounded by a toxic environment that affects our brains and our bodies. We pay little attention to the signs that we are influenced by these things. Maybe the constant allergies are from seasonal plants or maybe they are related to other environmental issues.

We have computer screens in front of our bodies for hours each day. Wireless internet waves constantly bombard us whether we are on the computer or phones. Radios, televisions, Bluetooth, sonar, and solar energy send signals through the air, the ground, and the walls. It is becoming impossible to escape all the quiet invisible noise.

Televisions, computers, video games, and cell phones consume your attention and drain your brain.

Take time, go outside, and look up. There is something there that you do not see all the time. Most of us look at the ground as we walk. Are you passing up the millions of things you could see, just to pick up pennies?

Observe the world in which you exist. When you are outside of your regular environment, do your allergies seem reduced? Are there some fabrics that induce rashes, or itching? How do detergents and soaps affect your skin? Are the reactions increased at certain times? Observe.

Your brain can read a temperature change of less than one degree. One moment you are comfortable and the next you are too warm or cold.

Clutter and knick-knacks collect more dust. Beyond thinking only of the dust, it means many places are filled with stuff. Stuff takes up your mental energy.

Reduce the clutter. Leave room for empty spaces, new thoughts, ideas and rest. Rest your brain from all the continued input that is both recognized and invisible.

Observe the changes that are evident in your daily life as they occur. Make conscious decisions to reduce the extras. See what happens when you look at less.

Color is an option. Different colors have different effects on brain stress. The brain gets tired when a color causes it to work all the time. Subliminal levels of visual input can be overwhelming and can eat up the capacity for new thoughts, planning and playing. Choose color carefully. Be aware of how color affects your comfort.

Find a chair that fits your body, supports your skeleton and allows your feet to fully rest on the floor. Observe the factors that affect how comfortable a chair is to sit in for an extended period of time.

Beds can be a tricky issue. How old is the mattress you currently sleep on? Is there more than one person sleeping on the mattress? If more than one person is regularly sleeping on the mattress, it will not last as long. If either of the people sleeping on the mattress is carrying extra weight, the mattress will fatigue more quickly.

Assess.

When purchasing a mattress, spend time in the store. With your partner or alone, make several visits. Try out all the different beds. Go back at a later time and spend time with all the beds again. Make lists and notes about what you like and dislike. You spend at least 33% of your life in bed.

Rest is vital to brain health.

Moment of Awareness

(Please take this page and make notes as needed)

Image of Self

We all have images of who we are and how we fit into our own lives. Changes may have occurred in the actual self, but not necessarily in the image. We may think nothing has happened and we are the same as we always were. Being able to separate the old from the new has challenges, for everyone.

This is the perfect opportunity to create a new image of self. Within the discovery of the self will be the development of new self-awareness. Take your time and plan on continuing this exploration for the rest of your life.

There may be pieces missing from the puzzle. As more pieces are added the brain has a clearer picture. This does not mean all the doors which have been closed will suddenly open. The bigger picture reveals new potential.

Writing and publishing this book was difficult. Telling everyone about my brain problems is terrifying. I have to trust that I will be okay and that people will still like me.

Moment of Awareness

(Please take this page and make notes as needed)

We Are Asymmetrical

We all have one larger foot, dominant hand, stronger eye, longer leg, etc. One millimeter of difference between left and right and we are falling. When it senses that we are falling, the brain kicks in the self-righting system. All is wonderful when the brain is healthy. When brain injured or brain tired, the system might be damaged or delayed and actual falling is more likely. Falling is brain consuming. On the other hand, when you fall it may mean you discovered a new way to proceed.

One of the advantages to imbalance is that it initiates movement. Movement can be a small step or a huge jump. Assess your speed. If we fall a millimeter it is not as difficult as falling to the ground, but it is still falling. There is still anxiety and stress. Finding clarity in postural balance reduces brain strain. Falling all the time requires a great deal of brain power.

One of the biggest fears we have is falling.

Falling and failing . . . are only one letter apart. We don't want to be considered failures.

The brain reads millions of bits of information in a second. Why do we assume it will not notice that we are asymmetrical? Why do we think it can be fixed?

There are some things that can't be fixed.

Moment of Awareness

(Please take this page and make notes as needed)

Balance, Posture and Movement

These are key elements for assisting in the return from brain fog. Each of these plays a silent role in the ability for the brain to function at a more capable level. We take them for granted. We assume we have them under control. We are using them as foundations for life. We don't think about them. We wouldn't know what to do with them if we did think about them. We don't discuss them either.

Look at both the big picture and the individual specific defined areas of concern.

Finding clarity in postural balance reduces brain strain. Falling all the time requires a great deal of brain power.

Balance

Balance is imperative. Finding it is illusive.

Balance is a huge subject. Assess balance in many areas of your life.

Being out of balance is exhausting.

Existing in a balanced environment quiets the neurological systems and gives room for peace.

There are so many areas affected by balance. We have balanced diets, balanced checkbooks, balanced lives between work and home, balanced emotions. There are many balances we assume and many we create.

Yet we still live out of balance and don't even know it, until we finally fall down. Just tripping might not be enough; it might have to be a giant tumble. While on the ground, stop and assess. Yes, you fell over because you are out of balance. Do you even know how to get up again?

Find a full-length mirror and a clipboard or two. Stand in front of the mirror and take a look at yourself. Look at your shape. The outer rim is okay to start. Find something you like and then find something else you like. Find something besides the cellulite and wrinkles.

Pick up one foot and balance for a moment. Observe the foot on which you are standing. This is probably your shorter side. Most people will not step up onto a longer leg. They will slide down onto the shorter leg. Falling to the short side first initiates   movement.

One millimeter difference is all that it takes to be shorter on one side.

The naked eye does not always detect a couple of millimeters.

Put the clipboard under the foot on which you are standing. Stand on both feet and look in the mirror again. Step off the clipboard and assess. Take the two clipboards and stack them under the same foot, look in the mirror, stop and assess. Step away from the stack of clipboards, stand in front of the mirror.

Do the same thing on the other side. Stop and assess. Walk away and do nothing. Try this again at another time. Make a note if there is one which provides a sense of more stability and balance for you. Each clipboard is approximately 4-6 business cards thick. Make a little heel pad with some business cards and wear it in your shoe for an hour or so. Take it out and assess. Did the pad make you feel more stable? Did it relieve pressure or reduce pain in your knees or hips? Did it make it worse? Observe.

The benefit to using business cards is the ability to change the number of cards incrementally. It empowers the person with brain issues to be aware and pay attention to small details. These changes continue to challenge balance, awareness to the overall weight distribution on the feet, and attention to comfort.

This shoe pad may make no difference in your life, or it may be a solution to postural issues you have been having.

Look for solutions which provide support and allow for

creative possibility at a reasonable price so you know if they are helping before investing funds. Understand that solutions are temporary. Once the brain has accepted the difference, there will be the need to look for another solution. There is a need to constantly provide the brain with novel stimuli.

Being able to control the variables presented to the brain allows for personal responsibility in the outcome.

Always expect the outcome to be within your ability to assess your brain function.

Fall less far. It only takes a millimeter to initiate movement.

Reminding the brain of the lost parts of the body requires slow, accurate movements with awareness and attention. This is more than getting one tight muscle to relax. It is organization of more than 650 muscles, 205 bones and all the remaining components in posture, balance and movement. Organization of the whole system takes the pressure and tension off of the one tight muscle that you assume is the point of all problems.

The skeleton is the base support system for the body. Think about your bones. Become aware of your bones. Pay attention to your bones. Look at bones so you know what yours look like. They are all formed for the function they perform. Draw strength from your bones. When you stand on them and use them, they give strength and stability to your core being.

Posture

Posture is more than "sit or stand up straight." This concept includes how we present ourselves to our friends, family and others. Posture includes how countries position themselves in the world for communication. Our posture is non-verbal evidence of how we are feeling, participating, and presenting ourselves in the world.

When all is well, there is upright posture with our heads held high. There is a sense of balance within the skeletal structure allowing movement and ease. There are appropriate spaces for the organs and tissues, to allow all to function with limited restrictions. Our brains need blood flow to oxygenate, repair and rejuvenate cells.

When posture is stooped and out of alignment and balance, falling and failing is imminent. There is compression on the internal organs, potentially limiting their ability to perform their required tasks. Imbalance and asymmetry in posture requires additional brain function, musculature contraction and psychological stress. Disease and stress are added to the already overwhelmed body and brain.

Posture is the stance we hold in stillness and *acture,* termed by Moshe Feldenkrais, is posture in movement. With all the articulations in the skeleton, there is evidence that humans were created with a high potential for large and minute movements. It is necessary to understand both.

Our posture is an external communication of the image we have of ourselves. It allows other people to ascertain an impression of who they think we are. It also presents areas for both groups that reduce or enhance the ability to communicate with trust and ease. We all have blind spots in our personalities we do not acknowledge and are only made aware of when someone else brings the area to light. These areas are present and displayed by subtle insecurities and can be portrayed through our body language. Feeling positive and experiencing happiness is depicted through a different posture than depression and sadness.

Posture is stacking the bones of the skeleton in an organized fashion to support the weight and movement of the body and head. As the structure gets taller, with each additional stacked bone, support from the foundation becomes more important. Each joint is specifically designed to accommodate the movement required in the particular location. The shape and size of each individual bone, muscle, and other soft tissue connectors form the human body and bring the shape and structure to functionally perform the tasks of daily living. When all is in an organized form, there is little stress on any one system. Then the immediate request for action can be complied with and performed with ease and less pain.

As posture comes closer to being organized, the brain finds easier pathways to function.

Movement

Movement is a key to unlocking the closed doors of the brain. It is with the attention to change that new neuro-pathways are developed and integrated in the nervous system. Start with something that you are able to work with at any time. Do something that you can do when and where you are. Develop strategies for moving in your chair or bed, or standing in line. Movement is life.

There are long, large, small, and short muscles. Each time a muscle contracts, it brings two bones closer together. The biceps brachii bends the elbow, bringing the forearm and the upper arm closer together. It is easier to engage the large muscles. There are many short small muscles along the spinal vertebrae. To contract these muscles the movements will be small.

There can also be spasm, increased muscle tone and contraction in the tiny muscles. Take time and make the smallest movements possible with attention to the tiny muscles along the spine and in other parts of the body. Change your trunk with small movements to target these small spinal muscles. If the muscle is a half-inch long, how big do you think the movement would be? Take your fingers about a half inch apart, then bring them closer together. This is the range of movement available in a muscle that short.

This is not easy. We have missed being trained to create small movements. We accept the way we move to be the only option. What other way to move is there?

Notice dancers. They have the same skeletal and muscular structures as we do. They train regularly using slow and subtle movements to develop use of the different articulations of the body. When the joints articulate, the muscles are able to contract and relax. Muscle contractions move the skeleton. The skeleton is the support system for posture.

Movements assist in the development of safety, security, and support.

Start with small easy steps to develop the pattern of learning. Once there is a pattern of learning information, it is possible to change.

Make a slow, beautifully connected movement and then rest. Repeat and rest.

Safety, Security, and Support

High on the list of human needs is safety. When the brain is traumatized, some of the safety net developed over the whole lifetime may be damaged.

This is a time for assessment and to develop and provide strategies for future action steps. Take time to add personal and environmental support during stressful experiences.

As you feel a sense of being supported, your clarity in thought becomes more easily available for new thoughts.

As you feel safer and less stressed, your thoughts will flow forward more easily.

As you feel more secure, your challenges become easier to meet.

Learn to appreciate your new self.

Part II

Feldenkrais Method and BrainEase

For the Rest of Your Life . . .

Many ask how long it will be before the memory will return. When will the pain be gone? When can I expect a total healing will occur?

There may be improvements, better days than others, and moments of glory when all works as well as possible.

There are areas that have been weakened and will need more support. There will always be holes, ruts, and dark areas that are not as easily accessed or even perceived by the brain issues group member.

Experiencing the maximum use for the longest possible time requires moments with attention to the details of the action as it occurs.

Do small actions regularly. Include them throughout each day. Find your favorites and mingle them with the ones you find difficult.

There will be days when you do nothing, and nothing happens. Too many days avoiding paying attention to anything and it becomes difficult to pay attention at all.

Falling into the abyss will lead to hours of floating around without direction and stability. This is initially a choice and then there is the point of no return. Many wander through life in the fog and think they are tuned into themselves and the world around them.

Pay attention to your pacing. It is beneficial to have more than one pace depending on the activity.

If you have been pushing yourself to produce at 110% and now you are comfortable at 80%, make it the new 110%. Find help to complete the remaining 30%. Make a list with your favorite tasks at the top of the list, do what you are capable of completing, and allow others to help fill the void.

Acknowledgment and acceptance that help is needed makes the changes in your life tolerable.

Find strategies to complete the obligations and routines filling your life. Add challenges to build new pathways and use more brain cells. Improve your balance, posture and movement.

How large is your vista? How do you imagine your future?

Group membership is open to everyone. You can join in one or more categories. Each person is affected by brain issues either personally or in their family or social circle. Take time, assess. To which category of membership do you belong?

About the Feldenkrais Method®

There are people who influence our lives. Many times we never meet them in person. Moshe Feldenkrais is one of these people in my life. Studying and training in his brilliant work has given me the background knowledge and learned skills to explore options as they arise. Moshe's method of improving posture, balance, and movement has given me confidence to live with more ease. It is difficult enough to walk through life experiencing reduced brain function. With limitations in available resources, navigating the maze of medical treatment, rehabilitation, and healing is daunting for everyone involved.

Moshe Feldenkrais developed a brilliant body of work providing a framework for people who experience the desire to change posture, balance, capacity for movement and improve overall function.

"Movement is Life. Life is a process. Improve the quality of the process and you improve the quality of life itself." Moshe Feldenkrais

Alan Fraser writes, "Feldenkrais Method: Difficult to explain, wonderful to experience a practical and scientific way of addressing aspects of movement we seldom even think about or worry about . . . until we have a problem."

Many people suffer with posture-related pain, reduction in movement, and dysfunctional habitual patterns. There are others who experience injury, illness, or misuse in their lives and are left needing to find paths to healing. The Feldenkrais Method® is a unique approach that educates the body to move and function during daily activities with more efficiency and comfort. Feldenkrais practitioners have been providing innovative sessions to a variety of people including Olympic athletes, performing artists, children and adults with brain injuries, office workers experiencing pain, and individuals who have a desire to improve the quality of their daily lives.

Each touch communicates with the brain, sending a message through the muscular-skeletal system to bring awareness to the possible movements and request a change. With patience, the brain processes the request and sends a response. In turn the response is reviewed and appropriate actions are taken, sometimes correct and sometimes not. If not, the request is sent again and the process continues. One of the marvelous principles of the Feldenkrais Method is the width and depth of movements, from large motor skills to minute and imperceptible motor skills. All the movements combine to make the whole picture. When the size of the muscles is considered, the size of the movement has to be relative. Some muscles deep along the spine, holding the vertebrae in rigid position, take very small movements to enhance the ability to create movement.

The human body uses multiple systems to function. The skeleton is a support system and frame for posture. The muscles contract to move the skeleton, protect the organs, and provide warmth. Both systems work together in millions of complex patterns throughout a person's daily life. Each person has genetic, habitual, and postural patterns which affect the weight distribution and balance of the head. As organization of the systems occurs, movements become easier, and balance and brain function improve.

Benefits of the Feldenkrais Method include:

- Building neuro-pathways
- Improving posture, flexibility, balance, and coordination
- Enhancing physical well-being
- Reduction of chronic pain, fatigue, stress, and muscle strain
- Increasing function in cases of orthopedic or neurological problems
- Refining skills for athletes, artists, executives, etc.
- Developing awareness, attention, and thinking ability
- Increasing confidence and self-esteem
- Connecting the neuro-pathways with gentle movement
- Expediting recovery from injury
- Utilizing a greater portion of the thousands of individual movements available in the human body
- Restoring a sense of dignity

Feldenkrais sessions are done with the student fully clothed and standing, sitting, or lying on a firm worktable. The practitioner gently touches the student to assist in creating exceptionally small movements to facilitate the student's awareness and stimulate natural learning. Each move in the lesson is part of a communication that Feldenkrais likened to dancing or conversation. Gradually the student becomes aware of how the muscles and skeleton are involved in part or as a whole in the common movements that are part of daily living. As the internal awareness and picture of the body becomes clearer there is overall ease.

Moshe Feldenkrais (1903-1984) was a scientist of physics, and of mechanical and electrical engineering, with a doctoral degree from the Sorbonne in Paris, France. He was also a student of Jigoro Kano (founder of judo) and became one of the first judo champions in Europe, and was the originator of the

first judo club in France. He was highly educated and well read in physiology, anatomy, and neuropsychology. He published many books on the Feldenkrais Method and on judo. His work has been carried forward by the International Feldenkrais Guilds and thousands of trained Feldenkrais practitioners worldwide.

For more information: www.Feldenkrais.com

30- to 60-Second Moments of Awareness
Learn to Learn

Guidelines to this method were developed by Moshe Feldenkrais. (1975)

*"Movement is life. Without movement
life is unthinkable." (MF)*

Moshe Feldenkrais wrote a booklet, "Learn to Learn," in 1975. In it, he outlined guidelines to his method of learning. In this section, I am honoring him and the impact his work has brought to my life and the thousands of others he has touched over the decades. I have included his guidelines in the quotes marked "MF." I have then added my own brief descriptions to clarify my insights.

These ideas are opportunities to observe ourselves and learn to play with the concepts presented. Take time to consider any insights that come forward in your life.

How do we bring something new into our system? How do we create new neuro-pathways and re-create patterns of movement we have lost? What are the important elements to bring new life to our brains?

1. <u>Do Everything Very Slowly. (MF)</u>

> *"Time is the most important means of learning. To enable everybody without exception to learn, there should be plenty of time for everybody to assimilate the idea of the movement as well as the leisure to get used to the novelty of the situation." (MF)*

It takes time for the request to be acknowledged in the brain, a response to be sent out with directions for action, and then for the appropriate structures to engage and action to be completed.

That is a perfect world.

> *"Fast action at the beginning of learning is synonymous with strain and confusion which, together, make learning an unpleasant exertion." (MF)*

The brain may require more than one request sent before it receives the input, and then a given movement may require several responses with directions for action before the appropriate structures engage in any part of the action to be completed.

Being in a hurry does not mean the outcome will satisfy the request. It takes time for the whole puzzle to come together and the pattern to become comfortable.

What is the hurry? You have time to learn something new or you can keep struggling with being incapable. You are not just relaxing a muscle. You are organizing a whole complex system to distribute the weight and reduce tension on one particular area. Reduce the parasitic exertion until the pattern has become easy and pleasant. Then add speed and resistance. You have to differentiate parts that are locked together before the fine small movement adjustments can occur.

2. <u>Look for the Pleasant Sensation (MF)</u>

> *"Pleasure relaxes the breathing to become simple and easy. Excessive striving–to-improve impedes learning."* (MF)

Take your time and look for the least amount of pain, the most comfortable position, and the new movement. Find parts and pieces of yourself that have been buried, lost or injured.

Becoming attentive to your self is a slow process of quiet observation. This is a challenge for brain issues group members. Trying something new and following the pathway of development is a brain-intensive moment.

If you think that you are capable of doing ten things at once, try just one thing at a time. Leave breaks for the rest time. Pay real attention to yourself.

3. Do Not "Try" to Do Well (MF)

> *"Trying hard means that somehow a person knows that unless he makes a greater effort and applies himself harder he will not achieve his goals. Internal conviction of essential inadequacy is at the root of the urge to try as hard as one can, even when learning." (MF)*

We are accomplished at trying. We have tried hard, tried everything, tried to . . . Did the try ever become reality? Trying means the completion has not occurred. It is still a work in process . Trying hard is an odd thought and experience.

> *"Learn to do well, but do not try." (MF)*

4. Do Not Try to Do "Nicely" (MF)

> *"Intent to do nicely when learning introduces disharmony." (MF)*

When achieving acknowledgment from others the need to perform becomes the prominent focus. When working with your brain, there should be attention to your independent self. Be kind. If the process begins a little disorganized and feels rough to start, that is all a good thing. Keep working with the details, find a time when there is a place to participate in comfort, chose something you are able to perform with ease, and then add a portion of the new information. Brain learning is happening, and each step is useful as a portion of another task in the process of creating new strategies.

With this process, soon you will have a huge repertoire of new and functional pieces that can be sorted and mixed to create a whole new activity. Taking a look at your family's and society's structures, assess how you were taught to be recognized. Teaching the brain may include a new way to be recognized. Assess your present need to be who you think society would like you to be. Also assess your ability to be this person with your present situation.

> *"An act becomes nice when we do nothing but the act. Everything we do over and above that, or short of it, destroys harmony."* (MF)

5. <u>Insist on Easy, Light Movement (MF)</u>

> *"We usually learn the hard way. We are taught that trying hard is a virtue of life, and we are misled into believing that trying hard is also a virtue when learning."* (MF)

Pushing hard, inducing pain, and forcing issues does not lead to a path of learning. It is difficult to learn something new when in trauma, stress, fast-paced existence, and pain.

> *"Learning takes place through our nervous system, which is so structured as to detect and select, from among our trials and errors, the more effective trial."* (MF)

Working with curiosity to find several options to a process allows the brain to make choices. When we act in a rote manner, living the assumption that the way we do it is the way it is done, we limit the potential outcomes.

> *"We sense differences and select the food from the useless: that is, we differentiate."* (MF)

We hurriedly take what is in front of us without looking around to find if this is the best situation for the particular moment and for our needs at the time. Maybe an additional moment of assessment would multiply the outcome benefits.

It may be uncomfortable to move slowly and be more observant. What happens if someone else gets the first spot? I like to think that maybe the second spot is more perfect for me. One large lesson is to locate experience and choose an easier path--for you.

6. <u>It Is Easier to Tell Differences When the Effort Is Light (MF)</u>

> *"All our senses are so built that we can distinguish minute differences when our senses are only slightly stimulated. In short, the smaller the exertion, the finer the increment or decrement that we can distinguish and, also, the finer our differentiation (that is, the mobilization of our muscles in consequence of our sensations). The lighter the effort we make, the faster is our learning of any skill; and the level of perfection we can attain goes hand in hand with the finesse we obtain. We stop improving when we sense no difference in the effort made or in the movement."* (MF)

Light effort is similar to the breath of wind on the back of the neck, a light touch on the skin, or a movement so minute that it is imperceptible to the observer and totally in the constant awareness of the participant.

There are small short muscles that are responsible for delicate movements. The size of the muscle determines the dimension of the movement. By standing and closing the eyes, paying attention to the neck and then moving the eyes from left to right, activation of the contractions of many small muscles in the neck may be felt. Shifting weight distribution by a gram or millimeter through the whole body will reduce or add to the strain on all the muscles and their capability to find and maintain ease in posture and balance. With the application of light pressure, a neuromuscular connection occurs and a greater potential to experience awareness of the differences is the outcome.

Transitioning from wide daily use of heavy gross motor movements can be simplified by integrating light fine motor movements throughout daily activities. Noticing change is a learned assessment skill.

7. <u>Learning and Life Are Not the Same Thing (MF)</u>

"In the course of our lives, we may be called upon to make enormous efforts sometimes beyond what we believe we can produce." (MF)

Life is a process, not an event. There are decisions that are made long before the outcomes are evident. Being able to surf the emotions, physical responses, mental traumas, and environmental issues is mandatory for everyone.

Those who fall sometimes find it too difficult to get up. They wonder who will save them. Why are they the chosen ones? What else can happen? These are questions that might be asked after the other million optional questions have been answered.

Brain issues group members are "called upon to make enormous efforts" to live their daily lives. Paying the dues and actively participating in life changes allows the sense of personal satisfaction and reduction in fear.

Society pays enormous dues to encounter and work with the all the people with brain issues. The message is to stay as healthy as possible. The system is straining with the multitudes of new members.

> "Learning must be slow and varied in effort until the parasitic efforts are weeded out; then we have little difficulty in acting fast and powerfully." (MF)

Parasitic efforts include all the extraneous movements and processes that hamper the direct functional path from beginning to end.

8. Why Bother to Be So Efficient?

> "We need not be efficient, because a kilogram of sugar yields roughly speaking 20,000 calories and one gram calorie produces 426 kilograms of work. From that count we can waste energy galore... The trouble lies in that energy cannot be destroyed; it can only be transformed into movement, or into another form of energy." (MF)

When posture causes the body to fall, we exhaust the mental freedom to create new thought. The energy necessary for clear thinking to occur has been utilized in the self-righting system. Even one millimeter of asymmetry causes the body to fall toward the shorter side. When there is efficient posture, balance and movement, we are less likely to experience aches, pains, and reduction in the activities we love.

Save your energy for great memory-making moments with neighbors, your family, and friends. Live a life full of movements, complete with many options, a sense of ease, and elegance. Make your brain smile.

9. Do Not Concentrate (MF)

"Attend well to the entire situation, your body, and your surroundings by scanning the whole of yourself sufficiently to become aware of any change or difference, concentrating just enough to perceive it. In general, it is not what we do that is important, but how we do it." (MF)

Working hard to concentrate is straining the brain; it begins by reducing the flow. Open your attention to take in the vista and the foreground at the same time. Pick up on colors, shapes, textures, and sounds at the same time. Then focus on something specific. Be able to move your attention between the two.
Severe concentration may create chaos in the function and ease of gathering thoughts. Lose anything, add the idea that you are already late, and there are three people talking to you at the same time.

Stop and assess. Let it go. Breathe.

10. <u>We Do Not Say at the Start What the Final Stage Will Be (MF)</u>

> *"By reducing the urge to achieve, and attending also to the means for achieving, we learn easier. Achieving—we lose the incentive for learning and, therefore accept a lower level than the potential we are endowed with. ... On knowing what to achieve before we have learned to learn, we can reach only the limit of our ignorance ... "* (MF)

Designing the outcome before the beginning forces the path in a certain direction. We are dealing with uncharted territory and have a preplanned map. There is a hole in this design model.

Learn something new every day. Participate every day. Say yes to activities. With all that this world has to offer, it would be a rare day when there was nothing to learn. Occasionally stay up late until you meet your goal for learning one thing every day. You will learn to start earlier in the day.

11. <u>Do a Little Less Than You Can (MF)</u>

> *"By doing a little less than you really can, you will attain a higher performance than the one you can now conceive. Do a little less than your utmost while learning. You are thereby pushing your possible record to a higher setting."* (MF)

Live challenging your boundaries and yet understand the value of living within your abilities.

Learn to live with less, doing less, and making less chaos in your daily life. Take the spare time that was consumed by your busy-ness and learn more that benefits you as a brain issues group member and the others in society around you.

12. <u>Some Useful Hints (MF)</u>

> *"Every now and then, do the exercise mentally only."* (MF)

> *"Lie still, or sit, and imagine your body performing all the movements. See yourself doing it in your mind's eye and note the mobilization of the skeleton and muscles "in the bud" so to speak, without gross apparent movements."* (MF)

Take time to mentally move through the patterns without physically participating. Each day take pieces of the movement patterns and do them from memory at least once. Do the sequences of movements throughout the day to make a habit of the patterns.

Transfer the concepts of learning to other areas of your life. Each area of your life improves with the new ability to assess and change patterns. Your physical, mental and emotional well-being will recover and develop with the newfound freedom of posture, balance, and movement in your life.

> *"Adjust to your capabilities."* (MF)

Do what you are capable of doing, and when you reach your limits, stop, hold, and breathe, and perhaps a small addition to the movement may be possible. Breathe again and slowly release the tension and desire to achieve. Attend to yourself. Improvement happens over time with patience and lack of effort.

> "Never overcome pain, if for some reason you feel pain." (MF)

Stop if the pain increases, slow down, do less. With slow small movements and gently repeating the action, greater range of movement happens.

Pain is a response that indicates injury is potential or has occurred. Tissue and joint damage creates irritation and inflammation, diminishing the healing process. Reduce the desire to continue to injure yourself. Making the movement of a circle with the shoulder can be a circle the size of the head of a pin or a basketball. All the movements are still circles involving the contraction and release of the same muscles.

> "Make your training a habit." (MF)

Find pleasure in the adventure faced each day. Take a small pattern and play with the optional movements over the process of a day or week. Make an appointment with yourself for your explorations and learning. Put it into your calendar to define it as important in your life.

Stop before the habit becomes a compulsion.

Because one movement feels great, be aware that making 100 rote movements with momentum does not make a learning process happen. It may only exhaust the systems and the outcome is reduced.

There are so many possibilities; there is no wrong movement.

It may be that you have moved too fast, used too much effort, or not organized the structures necessary to increase the range. There may be another movement in a sequence which has to occur in order to make the whole picture happen.

Seek guidance and assistance.

Find the best resources available to meet your personal needs.

Feel confident in yourself and your ability to learn.

Moment of Awareness

(Please take this page and make notes as needed)

30- to 60-Second Moments of Awareness Strategies for Daily Practice.

These are thirty-one opportunities to assist in training your brain. There is no specific order or length of time to use these. Consider using them for the rest of your life.

First Things First

1. Weight Through the Heels
2. Feet to Head
3. Feet Observing
4. Breathing
5. Head Toward Ceiling
6. Feet to Hips
7. Heel to Toe
8. Attention to One Side
9. Circles With the Nose
10. Eyes in Back of Head
11. Straight Arm Swinging
12. Balancing a Quarter on the Head
13. Laughing Daily
14. Nose to Neck
15. Swinging Arms--One Hand Pushing
16. Moving From Sitting to Standing
17. Tongue Between the Teeth
18. Finger Pressing-One at a Time
19. Building a Brain White Board
20. Step Backward

21. Open Your Eyes
22. Walking With Open Eyes
23. Climbing the Stairs
24. Balance on One Leg
25. Chewing
26. Rocking the Pelvis
27. Rolling the Feet
28. Grip--Move From Large to Small
29. Move From the Top of the Neck
30. Move From the Bottom of the Neck
31. Imagine

First Things First

Moments of Awareness are strategies for people with brain issues, which include simple ideas and explorations in movements for everyone to play with throughout the rest of their lives. Read, record, or have someone else read the exercises and slowly follow the concepts and movement processes.

Finding the stable support necessary for the brain to quit screaming, "Please help me, I'm falling!!!" is an acquired skill.

There are habitual patterns formed in the body prior to birth which affect our posture.

When posture supports the head, balance becomes easier. Assess your head position.

If you frame a house and put up four walls, making one wall six inches shorter than the other three, put the roof on top of the building and wait for a few decades, what happens to the structure over the years?

Which is your short wall? How much weight is the head on the structure? The head usually weighs between ten and twelve pounds. For every inch the head is positioned forward of the center line, add an additional ten pounds.

With the weight forward you are losing your balance. If you are asymmetric by one millimeter, you are falling. The self-righting system prevents us from completely falling.

Exhaustion to the systems occurs when there is falling all the time. There may be damage to the self-righting system. Falling may become more frequent. Balancing through the supporting skeleton is vitally important.

Support leads to a sense of safety, which leads to a space open for other tasks to occur.

First stage shock is the startle reflex of the infant. Second stage shock, which can occur at any age, is the fetal position to protect the vital organs. The head in the forward position when standing challenges the balance more than when lying in bed. It is difficult to find upright posture when the psychological and physiological response in the body is trauma. Layers of imbalance, from posture to life changes, compound the expectation on the brain.

Learning to unfold from trauma requires an environment and framework of safety, security, and support. Feeling vulnerable is not a simple experience to overcome. When noticing the changes occurring in your life there will be moments where fear and concern come forward.

Participating in these small movements may leave a sense of openness and freedom. If necessary, do them in private to be able to observe any physical and psychological differences that might arise. Many will be subtle, with the potential for being long lasting. Find a couple of minutes to let the movement settle into your system before moving on with your life.

Small muscles require small movements. Slow tiny movements may be necessary to initiate movement in chronically contracted small deep internal muscles. Large muscles on the outer layer of the body are easier to touch, activate and change.

Orientation is the position of the person: sitting, kneeling, standing, or reclining. Most of the movements are possible in all of these positions and it is beneficial to do all of them in the different positions.

Any and all of these are available to be incorporated throughout the day. Choose how you want to learn. Take one sequence and follow the instructions. Start with one or two times to several times a day. Do another one on another day. Just choose one and focus on the sequence for the whole day or a whole week.

When the car tire is in the rut, it took many trips to create the rut, many to get out of the rut, and many more to build a new rut.

We are training a brain. We are creating awareness to small direct movements that may have been forgotten and lost in the file cabinet of life. We are doing more than releasing a tight spot. It takes time for the brain to hear your request, perform the task of moving in a new pattern and meeting the criteria of the request, and then to memorize the new pattern. There may be several attempts that are off target and the response is not accurate.

If the task is easy to accomplish it is not one that needs to be learned. It is the difficult ones that are lost in our brain and have to be established again that we are seeking. Mix the easy with the difficult to appreciate how to refine the known and explore the lost.

Standing is balancing the whole body over the floor or other surface. A combination of flexibility and stability is required for the body as it adjusts to the environment. Most people have been doing it for their whole lives. But there might be a more efficient position.

Placing your feet about shoulder- or hip-width apart allows for a more solid base. Try them closer together. Try them further apart. Find a position and know that changing this stance is a learning opportunity. Do so frequently. The only stuck place is the inflexible brain.

Gravity is a two-way street; as we stand in posture as a reaction to gravity. We push up from the earth and pull down at the same time. The skeleton is the device the body uses to maintain shape against this force. Posture includes pressing down and pushing up at the same time. This is an activity of the subconscious brain; thank you, brain.

When lying, sitting, or standing, play with the padding used to support your legs, head, shoulders, or other parts for more comfort. Use cushions to pad your legs and feet when sitting in a chair. Put a small pillow under your shoulders when lying. Use only an inch or two under your head when lying. Put a heel pad in one shoe. Put a pad in the seat of your car to sit on. Observe and assess. Are you more or less comfortable? You are the one who is best able to assess your changes in comfort. It is common to accept the status quo and live with the outcome of pain. Change requires personal responsibility.

There are benefits to all of the thousands of movement patterns available in the human skeleton and muscular system. With a wide variety of patterns, balance, security, and support are easier to find and maintain. Being able to move from one to another is beneficial for long life with maximal lifestyle freedom.

Have patience as you start to make small changes in your life. There is a desire to have perfection within moments. First, appreciate the small steps of finding balance. Look forward to standing on the circus ball during the second day. Make the outcome achievable and pleasant.

These short movement sequences are designed to bring attention to a specific area during a small movement. They are not about releasing a single muscle; they are to assist in organizing all the structure to reduce the stress on any one area.

It is very important to take time to understand; observations of something new or different may not be remarkable or detectable.

If you are unable to commit 60 seconds of attention, wait until you can, or start with the 30-second sequences.

Attention and awareness for 30 seconds is not a simple task. Block out all but this moment and say "ahhhh" when complete.

For example, chose one side and pay attention to only one side for a whole day.

It is important to do something.

Who Will Benefit?

Everyone who has 30-60 seconds to experience a movement pattern with concentrated awareness will benefit. These movements are not created to release one tight muscle. They have been developed to organize the whole physical system to reduce the tension on one muscle. Take your time, reduce your effort, play with the concepts, quiet your mind and allow new information to enter.

Suggestions for Supplies

- Stool or chair
- Roller/fun noodle/can/rolling pin
- 6-8" Ball/4" ball - these are best if they are slightly soft.
- Walking sticks
- Wall
- Cushions
- Fabric shawl
- Clipboard
- Clothespin or refrigerator clips
- Coin
- Use other items in your environment. Find things that help to create small restrictions, challenges, or support movements.

Strategies for Success

Gather small items to pick up and touch that bring sensations or challenges to your brain.

Look around your home and office to find everyday items that you can utilize to enhance your neuro-pathways. Feel, hear, smell, see, taste.

Find things that work to create awareness in your life.

Challenge your brain to step outside your routine. A challenge may be as simple as pinching a clothespin between a new combination of fingers.

Develop strategies using parts and pieces that fit into the many puzzles of daily life.

Routines are built over time to get from point "a" to point "b." Strategies are pieces of the puzzle that are put together in different order to make a pathway from somewhere to another where. There are many pieces that are able to come together and make the pathway. Each time you are confronted with a new need, your brain is able to pull pieces together and create a strategy for the pathway. Strategies may become routines over time and use.

There is a benefit from experiencing each of these as individual processes. When two processes are comfortable there is a new ensemble when combined together.

Examples of ensembles include groups of movements, musicians, or articles of clothing; each is capable of being organized as an individual piece or working together in harmony.

When the movement is difficult it is a great one to work with more often.

Work in the privacy of your room if you would feel more comfortable. There is difficulty in having to produce a positive outcome when the subject or process is new.

Mistakes are great, something new to work with over time. Privacy is a great place to begin when feeling overwhelmed.

Do one pattern for a day or two and then play with a different pattern for a day or two. Be kind. No stress.

Each process includes statements of benefit, observations to enhance the experience, and cautions to reduce strain and overwork.

1. Weight Through the Heels

Standing: 60 seconds

Rest your hands, hand, or finger on something so the observation will be about posture. Work in stages; this is an observation of what is happening with your weight distribution during standing. Minimize the number of variables when beginning so concentration on a few things is possible. When working with this later, let your hand be free. This challenges your balance at the same time.

Place weight onto the heels. Return the toes to the ground. Let the heels sink into the floor. Slowly, slightly rotate your knees outward without moving the feet. Stand and breathe to allow the brain to find and file this moment. Slowly let go of this stance and notice what happens to the body. Repeat this process and note what occurs when the weight is placed on the heels and what happens when the pressure is released.

Stand and place weight onto the balls of the feet. Rest the whole foot on the floor with more pressure on the balls of the feet. Breathe and observe the comfort of this position. Do this with your feet with different widths of separation. Find which position offers the most support.

Benefit:

Build a sense of balance when standing, using the skeleton as a postural support system to build brain and body ease.

Observation:

Pay attention to when you sense support. Look beyond what you have made "comfortable" due to habitual patterns.

The difference between one position with weight onto the heels and the release of the pressure on the heels is the amount you are falling.

Notice any changes in the tension in the feet, legs, hips, low back, arms, hands, ribcage, neck and/or jaw.

Notice when turning the knees slowly there is a feeling of contraction in the buttocks and support of the pelvis.

You experience this tension all the time until you complete this moment of awareness and discover that there is an option.

Caution:

Place whole foot on floor, when pressing through heels; slowly shift weight without lifting toes.

Sink onto floor. Allow the floor to hold your weight.

Allow your knees to soften and bend slightly as the movement occurs.

It is only a mini movement when turning the knees.

2. Feet to Head

Standing: 60 seconds

Stand and rest your hands on something (wall, counter top, back of chair, grocery cart handle, table).

Begin by pressing onto the floor with the heels of the feet. Find the stable spot. Slowly begin to press up through the skull toward the ceiling at the same time.

To find the point of the head going to the ceiling, lightly tap the top of the skull to create a point of reference. Gently press down onto the feet and then slowly grow toward the ceiling.

Adjust the head position so that the top is moving upward with the eyes looking forward to the horizon.

Place your index finger lightly on the space above the lip and directly below the nose, slowly lower and lift the nose.

Place your index finger on the chin, slowly lower and lift the nose.

There are different outcomes to each one of these directions. Learning may occur in the brain with each one of these options.

Benefit:

Increase the movements in the neck and balance of the head while standing.

Observation:

If you see the ceiling, slightly lower the nose. If you see the floor, lift the nose.

I use the nose for reference because it is attached to the skull; the jaw is a separate bone structure.

Lengthening muscles that have been tight for years is a slow process. There is much to organize and learn to complete the task.

When you apply more effort in the system by pushing harder and increasing speed at the same time, be aware the outcome may be what you already know.

Make small adjustments as there is softness in the musculature of the lips, mouth, face, and throat to move into or with.

Caution:

Slow is "paint drying" slowness. Speed tightens the system and creates tension.

We are brain training; this is a "brain-iathalon."

When touching the upper lip area, engage the contact of the skin on both sides and sink into the soft tissue until you reach the solid structure underneath.

Be kind; it is your face.

3. Feet Observing

Standing or sitting: 60 seconds

Stand and rest your hands on something (wall, counter top, back of chair, grocery cart handle, table). Sit with feet comfortably flat on the floor.

Observe each foot individually. Is the pressure on the same places on both feet?

Observe each independent toe from great toe to the smallest toe. Number them one to five from great toe to smallest toe.

Observe which toes are holding tight and gripping. Observe the heels. Choose a foot.

During this sequence, rest and observe between each movement.

Move pressure in a small wave action from the heel to the smallest toe number five.

Move pressure in a small wave action from the smallest toe number five to the heel. Rest and observe.

Move pressure in a small wave action from the heel to toe number four.

Move pressure in a small wave action from toe number four to the heel. Rest and observe.

Move pressure in a small wave action from the heel to toe number three.

Move pressure in a small wave action from toe number three to the heel. Rest and observe.

Move pressure in a small wave action from the heel to toe number two.

Move pressure in a small wave action from toe number two to the heel. Rest and observe.

Move pressure in a small wave action from the heel to the great toe, number one.

Move pressure in a small wave action from toe number one to the heel. Rest and observe.

Move pressure from toe one to toe five to toe one.

Benefit:

Having feet to stand on with a broader spectrum of support and balance.

Observation:

Observe the pressure and tension in the foot at beginning and end of sequence.

Move slowly and hold the movement at the end of each sequence.

Caution:

Rest does not mean push.

4. Breathing

Standing, Sitting, or Lying: 60 seconds

There are many breathing patterns and suggestions which come from different cultures, studies and practices.

Oxygenation assists in the opportunity for clarity of the thoughts and activity in the brain.

Breathe often. Take time throughout the days, months and years to appreciate breathing.

Breathing starts with the diaphragm being in a position for contraction and release. This provides the ability for complete inhalation and exhalation. This comes from posture which allows the pelvis to align with the thoracic region.

The attachments of diaphragm connect from the low back around the bottom of the ribcage to front at the end of the sternum. When there is asymmetry there is tension in the diaphragm and the ability for function is reduced.

Finding the neutral pelvis to reduce the tension is the discovery. There may be as much as thirty degrees' difference in the angle of the female and male pelvis. This creates differences in the male and female breathing patterns.
While inhaling, the diaphragm contracts down allowing the lungs to fill and the ribcage to rise with the process.
While exhaling, the diaphragm releases, the lungs empty, and the ribcage falls.

Start with sitting and then transfer the information to orientations of lying and standing.

Sit on a chair or stool where you feel the two bones in your bottom. Place both feet on the floor with your weight on the heels to support your pelvis. If you are unable to reach the floor, put books under each foot until you are able to sit with comfort.

Place hands on waist and tuck the tail slightly under, and then move your pelvis so that you slightly stick your bottom out. Slowly move between the two positions. Find a point in the center where sitting is easy and breath is able to flow.

Notice your feet and knees. Are they apart or together? Try different combinations until you find ease in sitting and breathing.

Take a moment to pay attention to your current breathing pattern.

Do you inhale and exhale through your nose?
Do you inhale and exhale through your mouth?
Do you inhale through your nose and exhale through your mouth making a hoooo sound.
Do you inhale through your nose and exhale through your mouth making a haaaaa sound?

Each breathing pattern activates specific muscle patterns. Pay attention to each pattern as you take several breaths.

The inhale and exhale through your nose activate the muscles in the upper ribs and neck.
The inhale and exhale through your mouth activate the muscles in the face.

The inhale through the nose and exhale through the mouth making a hoooo sound activate the muscles of the anterior ribcage.

The inhale through the nose and exhale through the mouth making a haaaaa sound releases the diaphragm and other deep muscles attached to the lumbar spine allowing a stress and pain relief in the whole body.

Choose a breathing pattern for reduction in stress and pain.

Sit with feet on the floor. Observe the width between the knees. Do a sequence with the knees close together. Do another sequence with the knees very far apart. Do a series with the heels closer together and further apart. Observe the differences.

Find the place where the breath is full and easy.

Benefit:

Completing both inhalation and exhalation with ease and sense of fullness increases brain and physical ease. Expansion in the oxygenation and blood flow throughout the body feeds the nutrients necessary to support brain function.

Observation:

Those who breathe, live.

This breathing pattern calms the fight-or-flight response. Tension restricts breathing, trauma restricts breathing, and posture restricts breathing.

Finding the neutral pelvis to reduce the strain on the diaphragm is the discovery.

There are two bones on the base of the pelvis. These are designed for sitting upon to ease posture and maximize the ability to balance the head on top of the spine.

Observe the location of the pelvis to find the fullest breath. Take time in the space between breaths.

Use this sequence when stress or confusion in your daily life occurs.

Observe the difference between the exhalation through the nose or using the "haaa" sound and the exhalation using the "hooo" sound.

Caution:

Too fast or too far restricts the opportunity to breathe.

5. Head Toward the Ceiling

Standing or Sitting: 30 Seconds

Rest your hands on something.

Balance is not the primary attention.

Slightly rest with pressure through the heels onto the ground. Press through the heels. Try this with the knees slowly rotated outward and then with the knees rotated inward.

Put a coin on top of the head.
Push the coin on top of the head toward the ceiling.
Lengthen from the floor toward the ceiling through the skeleton from feet to head.

Expand with an up and down pressure at the same time. Hold and count to fifteen.

Complete a "soft" and "belly" breathing pattern (see no. 4, above).

Slowly release the tension of the expansion to reduce and maintain the lengthening that occurred. Continue to balance the coin on top of the head.

Benefit:

Pushing down and rising up at the same time lengthens the spine and creates a sense of posture, balance and greater availability for movements to occur.

Observation:

The force of gravity presses from top down and bottom down. Resist the force of gravity by pushing up and down against the pressure.

Hold the lengthened position and breathe.
Slowly release the tension.

Caution:

Fast and forceful will bypass the moment of meeting the gravitational force, and stiffness will occur.

Head-forward posture has more difficulty with carriage of the coin.

Long-standing patterns of posture take more than sixty seconds to change.

5. Feet to Hips

Sitting: 60 seconds

Sit with feet flat on the floor in front of you. Bring the feet and knees together side by side. Press gently onto the balls of your feet together at the same time and hold the pressure. Count six seconds. Breathe in and continue to hold the pressure. On the exhale, slowly release the pressure on the balls of the feet.

Rest through an inhalation and exhalation of the breath cycle. Place the pressure onto the heels of both feet at the same time and hold the pressure. Count six seconds. Breathe in and continue to hold the pressure. On the exhale, slowly release the pressure on the heels of the feet.

Rest through an inhalation and exhalation of the breath cycle.

Move each foot until the space between the feet and knees is about six inches. Follow the directions above.

Move each foot until the space between the feet and knees is about twelve inches. Follow the directions above.

Move each foot until the space between the feet and knees is as wide as possible and still comfortable. Follow the directions above.

Benefit:

Working with distances between the feet and the effect on the legs and hips when sitting.

Observation:

Where are the feet and knees when beginning?
Are they together or apart?
Where is the pressure on each individual foot?
Which position is the most comfortable?
When you end, are your feet and knees in the same position as when you began?
What happens in the low back when applying pressure in the heels or the balls of the feet?

Caution:

Feet need to be flat on the floor. If the chair is too tall for that, make a platform for your feet with books, boxes, etc. Find a height that is tall enough to be comfortable.

Move slowly; add pressure by small increments.
Make the pressure effortless.
Apply pressure without tension.

When you move the pressure to the heels of the feet, hold the pressure and count slowly. Breathe and release slowly.

6. Heel to Toe

Sitting: 30 seconds

Begin with the feet together on the floor.

Place weight on the heel of one foot and the weight on the ball of the other foot, heel and ball. Hold the weight and count to ten.

Release slowly, allow the feet to rest on the floor and count to ten.

Change feet width and place the weight on the heel of the opposite foot and on the ball of the opposite foot. Hold the pressure and slowly count to ten.

Release slowly while counting to ten.

Benefit:

Increase the functional use of the ankles and feet to improve balance and support when standing.

Observation:

Place approximately the same amount of pressure on each foot at the same time.

Gradually increase the pressure after the initial contact begins. When the pressures become obvious, hold and begin the count.

Note which foot you chose to place weight in the heel first.

Go through the process when standing while placing hands on wall or counter. Slowly lift one heel, a small distance from the floor with the other foot on the ball and then move the pattern to the other foot.

Caution:

Take time to move slowly into the point of pressure and take time to release the pressure. Both directions are important.

Note the side of the body with the weight in the heel. What happens to the low back? What happens to the abdomen?

7. Attention to One Side

Walking: 30 seconds

Walk either from the house to the car, across a parking lot, in the mall, or in a hallway at work. Find a place where walking is easy and there nothing to step or trip over.

With each left foot as it lands say or think "**left**." Make the emphasis to the left foot only.

Left, left, left. Pay attention to the left leg and foot.
Left, left, left. Pay attention to the left side of the body.

Continue this for twenty seconds.

Keep walking without the "left" thought and emphasis, for ten seconds.

Stop for a moment and assess any differences.

Benefits:

Increase awareness of the difference between the two sides, determine which is more familiar and functionally create more balance in posture and ease in brain function.

Observation:

The more clear the focus, the greater the outcome.
Focus on what happens when the emphasis on the left side ends.

Caution:

Walk as you always walk. The focus is to bring awareness to an area that may not have been in the forefront.

Making a neuro-pathway requires the area of interest to be in the forefront of attention.

Change occurs when there is repetition of a pattern with attention to the process.

Pacing allows the brain to read the request and respond.

8. Circles With the Nose

Standing, Sitting or Lying: 30 Seconds

Rest your hands on your face with the palms on the chin, the thumbs along the bottom of the jaw and the fingers slightly spread.

Make a small circle with the nose. Slowly make the circle again making it round. Make the circle smaller and more accurate.

Stop and rest.

Begin to make the circle in the opposite direction.
Move slowly and be accurate in the roundness of the shape.

Make the circle slightly larger.

Stop and assess.

Take your hands away from the face and make the circle.

Observe the difference.

Benefit:

Engaging the musculature of the neck and face during the rotation of the nose to reduce tension and increase the functional use of the eyes and ribcage.

Observation:

There are over one hundred muscles in the neck.

Gently rest the hands on the face.

The head is not a pimple.

Observe the initial direction of the circle.
As the circle arcs around, notice if there are places where the arc disappears and a line happens.

Make the circle small. Learn to make the circle the size of the head of a pin. It is more important to make the circle in a round shape. Play with the concepts. Enjoy.

The circle can be made larger as the circle becomes round.

As the circle with the nose is being made it engages the muscles of the neck in contraction and lengthening.

If the movements are difficult, make them in your imagination. Make them slowly and picture a round circle when making the movement.

Caution:

Observe the speed. There is no competition for fastest circle.

The hands allow the weight of the head to be supported while the action of making the circle occurs.

Resting the elbows near the chest may assist in the process.

9. Eyes in Back of Head

Standing, Sitting or Lying: 60 seconds

Rest hands on face with thumbs toward ears and fingers spread on cheeks. Light holding and support is the goal.

Place imaginary eyes on the back of the head. Open and close these eyes slowly a couple of times.

Open the eyes on the back of your head and look out. Slowly look to the left. When you look to the left as far as comfortable, stop and close your eyes. Rest.

Open eyes on the back of your head and look out. Slowly look to the right. When you look to the right as far as comfortable, stop and close your eyes. Rest.

Benefit:

Reduce the limitations to vision and eye function beliefs and reduce the strain and tension of "looking" with intention.

Observation:

Rest hands gently as a support for the weight of the head.

Move slowly to pay attention to the back of the head in motion.

Make the movements with the eyes open.

Make the movements with the eyes closed.

Take time to visualize the environment that is present to the eyes in the back of the head.

Create an arc movement while looking from side to side.

Caution:

Stop when the movement becomes the front of the head instead of the back of the head.

Move slowly to allow time to see how to make movement from an unfamiliar location.

Rest with eyes open.

Rest with eyes closed

Take time to orient when returning to eyes in front of head.

10. Straight Arms Swinging

Walking: 60 seconds

Walk with your arms relatively straight at the elbow and when swinging forward the thumbs are upward toward the sky or ceiling. Swing both arms along each side of the body in a line with the body, not across the body.

Start with a small swing that synchronizes with the walking leg (right foot, right hand and left foot, left hand). Walk this way for 30 seconds.

Rest.

Change the synchronization to the opposite hand and foot swinging (right foot, left hand and left foot, right hand). Walk this way for 30 seconds.

Rest.

Benefit:

Experience the difference between unilateral and bilateral arms swinging in relationship to the legs. The expanded use of lateral and bilateral patterns assists in the functional use of both the left and right side of the brain.

Observation:

Notice there may be more comfort when walking in some of the different patterns. Pay attention to which pattern is easier for you. Move between the patterns more often.

Start with a small swing of the arms, notice where the movement occurs in the back.

Make the swing larger, notice where the movement occurs in the back.

Caution:

Walk slowly at first to allow the pattern to occur.

Keep the arms relatively straight with the hands flat and straight.

Keep the swinging arms in line with the body.

Keep the arms parallel to each other.

11. Balancing a Quarter on the Head

Walking, Sitting, Standing: 60 Seconds

Place a quarter on the top of your head.

Stand and balance the quarter.

Sit with the quarter.

Walk with the quarter.

Pick up the quarter when dropped and start again.
Feel the quarter sitting on top of your head.
Take the quarter off.

Do you still feel the quarter on top of your head?

Benefit:

Increase the sense of balance with the use of weight to allow the body to organize itself in upright posture while standing or sitting still and in movement patterns.

Observation:

Find the weight of the quarter to be noticeable.
Notice the movements that occur in the body to balance the quarter.

Do other coins provide the same effect?

Caution:

You may have to pick up the quarter many times.

13. Laughing Daily

Sitting, Standing, Lying: 30 seconds

Find a place to laugh. Find many places to laugh.
Think about a time when you laughed because something was funny.

Listen to the sound fill your memory.
Find the way your body reacts to the sound.
Look at what happens to your breathing.

Do you have a memory strong enough to start the laughing again?

Hold the laughter and let it build.
Live in the memory for a moment.
Slowly let the laugh slip out.

Hold the laugh from slipping out.
Make the memory more clear.

Where does the laughter begin in your body?
When you let the laugh escape what path does it take?

30 more seconds

Find something that happened today.

Make laughter about this incident.

Change the frustration into humor.

Laugh at yourself, with yourself and for yourself.

Benefit:

Joy in the brain. Physiological ease in all the systems, and happy people.

Observation:

Laughter happens when there is something light hearted.

Children laugh hundreds of times a day. Adults laugh fewer than ten times a day.

Do you only laugh when the outcome is pain for another person or animal?

Caution:

Find laughter with pleasant outcomes.

Laughter begins more laughter.

Laugh often.

14. Nose to Neck

Standing, Sitting or Lying: 30 seconds

Find the supported posture position.

Gently place tip of the index finger on the space under the nose and above the lip.

Slowly look down your nose and lower chin.

Slowly look upward and bring the chin to neutral.

Pay attention to the lengthening and shortening of the neck in the back.

Benefit:

Connect the nose to the upper neck and the skull to ease balance of the head and reduce the tension and holding patterns of the head, neck, jaw, and face.

Observation:

Move slowly to notice when the back of the neck gets longer.

Notice when the back of the neck gets wider.

Notice what happens in the neck where the head rests.

Notice what happens at the bottom of the neck.

Caution:

Go slowly.

Move in a range that is pain free.

If pain occurs, move slower and in a smaller range.

15. Swinging Arms – One Hand Pushing

Walking: 60 seconds

Walk with arms relatively straight at the elbow with the palms facing behind the body. The back of the hand will be toward the front of the body.

Swing both arms along each side of the body in a line with the body, not across the body.

Choose one hand and push the air from front to back during the swinging of the arm. With each swing push the air using only one arm.

Walk this way for 30 seconds.

Switch arms.

Benefit:

Application of pushing is similar to adding weight to the movement of the arm. The focus on one side increases awareness of the connections of the arm to the other parts of the body.

Observation:

Pushing air means taking air in the palm of the hand, from the front of the swing and pushing it past the body to the back and away.

Caution:

Push air with only one hand at a time.

Walk with ease.

Chose a walking pace that is comfortable and easy.

16. Moving From Sitting to Standing

Sitting: 30 Seconds

Sit comfortably with both feet flat on the floor.

Place one foot ahead of the opposite foot in a step pattern.

Place hands on thighs, toward the knees.

Place fingers on the outside of the thighs and the thumbs toward the inside of the thighs.

Put weight into the heel of the foot that is in the back position.

Slowly push down onto the thighs with the hands, lean forward and look upward while pushing weight onto the feet.

Begin to lift your bottom off the chair.

Scoop the bottom underneath the body and push through the heels to come to standing upright.

Switch feet position and stand in the opposite direction.

Benefit:

Creating ease in the transition from sitting to standing and standing to sitting. Being able to move from sitting to standing regardless of which direction the chair faces or side of the bed one is rising from.

Observation:

Sit slightly forward on the chair.
Using the hands to push on the thighs places the hands in a forward position instead of behind on the arms of the chair.

Use a slight rotation in rising if that is more helpful.

Work with different placements of the feet and find one that works best for you.

Leaning forward and looking up at the same time helps with momentum to rise from the chair.

Trade legs and become able to lift off the chair in either direction.

Caution:

When you look down it makes it difficult to get up.
Keep feet relatively close together. Avoid a wide stance from side to side or front to back.

When learning this, find a chair that has a firm seat for support.

17. Tongue Between the Teeth

Sitting, Standing or Lying: 30 seconds

Gently place the tip of your tongue between your teeth.

Hold the tongue lightly and gently with the teeth.
Slowly, count to ten out loud.

Articulate the words carefully and concisely.

Benefit:

Organize the tongue, face, jaw and neck with specific restrictions.

Observation:

Notice the ease in some numbers.

Feel the small movements of the tongue.

Articulate all the letters of each number slowly.

Caution:

Light pressure on the tongue.

Biting will hurt.

18. Finger Pressing, One at a Time

Sitting: 60 seconds

Rest your hands on a smooth firm surface.

Spread your fingers and lay palms on the surface.
Slowly press the index (first) finger onto the surface.
Inhale and increase the pressure. Hold the pressure.
On the slow exhale, release the pressure slowly.

Rest.

Slowly press the middle (second) finger onto the surface.

Inhale and increase the pressure. Hold the pressure.
On the slow exhale, release the pressure slowly.

Rest.

Slowly press the ring (third) finger onto the surface.
Inhale and increase the pressure. Hold the pressure.
On the slow exhale, release the pressure slowly.

Rest.

Slowly press the little (fourth) finger onto the surface.
Inhale and increase the pressure. Hold the pressure.
On the slow exhale, release the pressure slowly.

Rest.

Slowly press the thumb onto the surface.
Inhale and increase the pressure. Hold the pressure.

On the slow exhale, release the pressure slowly.

Rest.

Slowly press the heel of the hand onto the surface. Inhale and increase the pressure. Hold the pressure. On the slow exhale, release the pressure slowly.

Rest.

Benefit:

Make connections between the individual fingers, through the hands, wrists, elbows to the shoulders and neck. Reduce the strain and tension in the fingers, hands, wrists, elbows, shoulders and neck.

Observation:

Take a long slow inhale and long slow exhale.

Find the small space between each direction of the breath.

Release the tension in the pressure in the finger slowly with the breath.

Allow space between the changes in fingers to allow the tension to release.

Caution:

Move slowly into and out of the pressure.

19. Building a Brain Whiteboard or Screen

Sitting, Standing, Lying: 30 Seconds

Take a moment, close your eyes. Look at the space in front of your eyes. Think of it as an empty screen or whiteboard.

Think of a picture of something and place it on the board. Write the word that describes the picture on the board. Erase the picture and leave the word.

Find time to put words on the board. Do math problems on the board. Place pictures on the board. Take them away and put new pictures on the board.

I have used this board when I stumble on something in my conversation. I see the word that I am having difficulty pronouncing and then I am able to read the word.

Benefit:

Engaging a tool for brain-tired, -fogged, or -injured people to assist in moments where words escape and there are blank spots that can be filled with pictures, colors, patterns or words.

Observation:

Take time when there is a space for quiet.

Bring up one word, one picture, or one sound at a time and put them on the board. Take only one image and make it real, colorful, and accurate. Be able to erase the picture and leave the screen.

Take time to activate the screen and leave it alone. Find ways to make it useful in your daily routine.

This tool can become as small or large, colorful, pictured, lettered as desired or imagined. Engage the brain in creating and using a personalized tool as an option to blank moments.

Use it as needed when there is a blank stare and the words or ideas are difficult to pull forward.

Caution:

Use the screen when you have time to activate the possibilities.

Take time to rest often during this activity.

20. Step Backward

Walking, Standing: 30 seconds

Rest your hand on the wall, grocery cart handle, railing, or the hand of a friend.

The assistance will allow you to observe walking instead of struggling with balance.

Make the width of the backward step short and easy.
Rest the tip of the great toe on the floor.
Roll to the ball of the foot.

Roll until the whole foot is resting on the floor.
Place weight onto the heel.
Slowly, in a small movement, slightly rotate the knees out.

Lengthen the low back; bring the tail between the legs.

Slowly contract the abdominal muscles. Inhale slowly through the nose and then exhale through the mouth using the **"haaaa"** sound.

Balance.

Rest.

Find the balance to lift the opposite foot off the ground and stand on one foot.

Slowly place the lifted foot back on the ground.
Stand on both feet again.
Assess.

Benefit:

Stepping backward alters the balance and posture from falling forward to more upright. Without the use of the eyes the sensory system engages. This is the opposite of the habitual pattern of stepping forward and engages the whole body in different movements and brain pathways.

Observation:

Use the suggested support.

Move slowly.

Roll the foot slowly from tip of toe through to the heel.

Observe the movement of the pelvis and low back.

Take the time necessary for whole body to adjust during the process.

Move slowly to find the balance point for ease in lifting the leg.

Observe the length of time the leg is lifted.

Make up to four steps backward and then walk forward. Observe.

Caution:

The support is there to allow movement without visual orientation.

The use of the flexor muscles of the anterior body have to change jobs with the extensor muscles of the posterior body. This takes time when it is a new pattern.

Change the pelvis position and observe the ease in balance.

21. Open Your Eyes

Standing, Sitting or Lying: 60 seconds

Look out of your eyes.
Notice what you see.
Notice the boundaries of your vision while holding the head in a forward position.

Rest your hands on your face to support your head.
Gently hold your head in forward position.

Close your eyes.

Move your eyes to the right.
Move your eyes to the left.
Move your eyes upward.
Move your eyes downward.
Open your eyes and assess.
Gently move your head to the right and hold.

Close your eyes.

Move your eyes in the four directions.
Return your head to forward position.
Open your eyes and assess.
Gently hold your head to the left.
Move your eyes in the four directions.
Return your head to forward position.

Open eyes and assess.

Gently hold your head looking up.
Move your eyes in the four directions.

Return your head to forward position.
Open eyes and assess.

Gently hold your head looking down.
Move your eyes in the four directions.
Return your head to forward position.

Open eyes and assess.

Gently hold your head in forward position.
Close your eyes.

Move your eyes into the distance. Look very far.
Bring the eyes back to look behind you into the distance.
Bring the eyes to neutral.

Open eyes and assess.

Benefit:

Movement of the eyes is connected to the movement of the head and can restrict movements of the neck, ribcage, arms and hands. Moving the eyes in synchronized and differentiated patterns from the movement of the head increases the peripheral vision and reduces the strain in the connected areas of the body.

Observation:

Move quietly and slowly.
Assess differences between beginning and end in the boundaries of your vision.
Do a portion of the movements at any time.
Do restful eye movements prior to sleep.

Caution:

GO SLOW!
Eyes are busy almost all the time.
Eyes see light through the lids when closed.

22. Walking with Open Eyes

Walking: 30-60 seconds

Glance at the pathway in front of you. Look into the distance for anything that might cause you to stumble.

Walk with your eyes open looking into the distance.
Stop and stand.

Walk with your head down, looking at the ground in front of you.
Stop and stand.

Walk with your eyes scanning the distance.
Find an ease in walking with your eyes scanning the distance.

Move your gaze between the distance and close.

Benefit:

Walking with wide-eyed vision increases the ease of balance and reduces the tension in the hands, arms, shoulders, neck and face. Directing and tightening the vision increases the tension and tightens the musculature and increases the forward falling and fight-or-flight response.

Observation:

Notice what happens to your balance when walking with the gaze on the distance.

Notice what happens to your balance when walking and your vision is close and toward the ground.

Caution:

Observe the ground to avoid tripping.

Do this in a safe place, and then walk on a more uneven surface to challenge yourself when walking.

23. Climbing the Stairs

Standing: 60 seconds

Walk toward the stairs.
Look up the stairs.
Notice the landing, width, height, and railings.
Assess the climb.

Place one foot on the first stair.
Look up the stairs while climbing.
Use the handrail for support.

Transfer weight onto the stair.
Step back down onto the floor.

Step onto the stair; prepare to shift weight onto the next step.
Look down at the stairs and step up one stair.

While transferring weight from one step to the next, press through the foot when lifting onto the stair.

Benefit:

Increase the ability to transfer weight while climbing or stepping higher, with more ease and sense of balance.

Observation:

Notice when there is a point where it is possible to transfer weight easily.
Observe when the climb becomes more difficult.

Caution:

Plant the foot, place weight and then press through the foot.

Move up and down the bottom stair or two.

When there is ease on the first few steps, move up and down several stairs until the all the stairs become easy.

24. Balance on One Leg

Standing: 30-60 seconds

Find a comfortable place to stand.
Place your hand on the wall, counter, table, or chair.
Prepare to step slowly backward.
Place the tip of a toe on the ground.
Roll through the ball of the foot to the heel.
Place weight onto the foot with pressure on the heel.
Push the head toward the ceiling.
Engage the abdominal muscles.
Balance.
If you are comfortable, take your hand away from the support.
Use the breathing pattern of inhalation through the nose, exhalation through the mouth using the **"haaaa"** sound.
Slowly lift the opposite foot and leg.
Stand and hold.
30 seconds . . . 60 seconds . . .
Slowly lower foot to the floor and rest standing over two feet.
Assess.
Change the balance process to the other foot and leg.

Benefit:

Change the functional use of the anterior and posterior muscles from flexors to extensors. Increase awareness of posture and ability to maintain support while balancing on one leg.

Observation:

The length of time you are able to balance on one foot.

Observe balance when eyes are open.
Observe balance when eyes are closed.

Caution:

Take time to balance.

If at any time you feel as though you might fall, return hand to supporting wall, counter, table, or chair.

Be kind. Stand on one leg for as long as possible. It may begin with the initiation of lifting the foot and leg and using imagination to stand on one foot.

25. Chewing

Sitting or Standing: 30 or 60 seconds

Sit with a small plate of food.
Notice the aroma of the food.
Look at the texture.
Look at the color.

Place a small bite of food into your mouth.
Hold the food on your tongue.
Chew slowly with your front teeth.
Assess the flavors and textures.
Take several seconds to chew and then swallow.

Sit quietly and breathe.

Take another small bite of food into your mouth.
Hold the food on the tongue.
Chew slowly with the teeth on the right side of your mouth.
Assess the flavors and textures.
Take several seconds to chew and then swallow.
Sit quietly and breathe.

Place a small bite of food into your mouth.
Hold the food on your tongue.
Chew slowly with the teeth on the left side of your mouth.
Assess the flavors and textures.
Take several seconds to chew and then swallow.

Sit quietly and breathe.

Benefit:

Happy, nutritionally supported body with functional use of the jaws, tongue, and neck to ease muscular tension, improve speech, and sense of smell.

Observation:

How does the food smell, look and taste?

Which side of your mouth is more comfortable when chewing?

Do your teeth have the same comfort on each side?

How does your tongue work to move the food in your mouth?

How fast or slow do you chew your food?

Caution:

Chew slowly to break the food down to a smaller size and allow the brain and body to better process the food.

26. Rocking the Pelvis

Lying: 60 seconds

Lie on your back with your knees bent and feet a comfortable distance apart, about the same width as the hips. Find the width where there is enough space between the knees and feet to be comfortable. Lay your head on a thin cushion for support.

Rest your arms comfortably away from your sides. Allow arms to roll, turning the hands to palms-up position.

Slowly lift the lower back by arching away from the surface. Make the movement slow and easy, then stop, holding in the air for the count of five. While exhaling, slowly lower your back to the original position.

Slowly lower the back so the waist is touching the surface you are lying on, by rolling the hip and slightly lifting the tail feathers toward the ceiling. Make the movement slow and easy. Stop where there is the beginning of pain. Inhale and hold the breath for a count of five, and while exhaling, slowly allow your back to come to a neutral position where there is no effort in either direction.

Repeat the sequence while breathing, alternating between slowly arching the back and lengthening the back, rocking the pelvis forward and backward. Each movement is slow, easy and pain free. Rock the pelvis slowly, like a pendulum swinging. Be kind and rest.

These movements can be completed in sitting, lying and eventually standing positions to ease the tension and holding patterns of the pelvis. Using inhalation and exhalation enhances the ability to complete the movement and bring more clear balance to the pelvis, low back and abdominal areas.

Benefit:

To create more balance between the lower back and abdominal area for postural ease and support when sitting, standing, or walking. Balance the weight of the trunk and head over the pelvis and legs for ease in posture and to increase mobility.

Observation:

Take time to lift your bottom slowly away from the surface.

As your bottom lifts, slightly contract the abdominal muscles.

Breathe.

Slowly return your bottom to the surface.

Notice the position of your feet.

Take note of the pressure in your legs and neck.

Caution:

Start with lifting your bottom an inch. As time passes, lift a little higher.

If there is stress in your neck, place a pad under your back and shoulders to just below the neck, to give room for the head and neck to reduce tension.

Move slowly in both directions.

27. Rolling the Feet

Sitting: 60 seconds

Sit with your feet on the floor.

Find a foam roller, rolling pin, can, or ball.

Place one foot on the object and keep the other foot on the floor to stabilize and support the body.

Gently begin to roll the foot over the surface of the object. Bring the heel of the foot toward the floor.

Roll the foot across the object so that the toes go closer to the ground.

Do this several times without pushing or pressure. Keep enough contact with the bottom of your foot so that you are able to feel the surface of the object. Sit tall so there is no pressure from leaning on the foot resting on the object.

Make the movement easy and comfortable.

Think of brushing the heel on the floor and then across to the other side, and think of touching your toes to the floor. It is not important to ever touch the floor. This is a see-saw movement.

Stop, take your foot off the object and let your foot rest on the floor.

Return your foot to the object.

Roll the outside of your foot back and forth, slowly.
Roll the inside of your foot back and forth, slowly.
Roll the foot around or over the object.

Rest. Take the foot to the floor.

Do other foot in the same pattern.

Benefit:

Softening the tension in the ankles, feet and legs to improve balance when standing and walking.

Observation:

Roll the feet slowly. Give time for the ankle to make the movements.

Control the object with your foot.

Be gentle with your feet.

Assess the foot while standing when completed with each side.

Caution:

Go slow.

Roll with as little tension as possible. Rolling and pushing are two different things.

28. Grip--Move from Large to Small

Sitting, Standing or Lying: 30-60 seconds

Choose a group of four to five balls of varying sizes from about four inches down to one inch.

Start with the largest ball you can hold in one hand and squeeze with ease. Over time move from largest to smallest ball.

Hold the ball in the palm of your hand. Have your palm facing up. Wrap your fingers around the ball.

Grip slowly and hold the ball snugly.

Put more pressure in the first finger. Hold for a few seconds. Release.

Put more pressure in the second finger. Hold for a few seconds. Release.

Put more pressure in the third finger. Hold for a few seconds. Release.

Put more pressure in the fourth finger. Hold for a few seconds. Release.

Put more pressure in the thumb. Hold for a few seconds. Release.

Open fingers slowly and let the ball sit in the palm of your hand. Rest.

Wrap the fingers around the ball gently.
Roll the hand over, palm down, and follow the directions for palm up.

Let the fingers open and release the ball.

Rest.

When you are comfortable with the smallest ball, move to more refined grasp and holding patterns. Place a few kidney beans in a bowl and pick them up with any two-finger combination. Move from large to small--kidney beans, lentils, and then grains of rice.

Benefit:

Use of fine motor skills and musculature of the fingers, hands, and wrists to engage the approximately twenty-five percent of motor neurons in the brain which are dedicated to the function of the hands.

Observation:

Notice which of your fingers are more able to apply pressure with ease.

Notice which of your fingers are stiff.

Notice how the whole hand feels when the ball is released and resting in the palm.

Notice how the whole hand feels when the hand is empty.

In time, you can do both hands at once.

Caution:

Assess when to move from one ball to the next size smaller. There is no rush. Become totally comfortable with the first size before moving to another size.

Occasionally move back to the larger size to assess the changes.

29. Move the Top of the Neck

Sitting, Standing or Lying: 30 seconds

Gently rest your hands on your face. Place your thumbs toward your ears and spread your fingers on your cheeks. Hold your head lightly.

With your head and face, slowly make the movement up and down like "MMM" across from left to right and right to left.

When making the movement, slowly lift and lower your chin. Pay attention to your chin during the movement.

Pay attention to the movement happening at the base of the skull.

Make the movement small.

Rest.

Benefit:

Connect with the support of the hands touching the face. Reduce the strain to the lower part of the neck and upper ribcage and ease the tension across the shoulders and down the arms using small movements of the neck.

Observation:

Where does the movement happen in the neck?

What happens when you remove your hands from your cheeks and do the movement without support?

What happens if you hold the head tightly?

How large of a movement do you make?

Caution:

Assess the speed and size of the movements.

How large are the muscles at the top of the neck along the spine and skull? How large do the movements need to be to activate a muscle that is less than an inch long?

Rest often.

Move slowly and notice where the movement originates and where the movement translates.

When you lift the chin slowly it is easier to access movement at the top of the neck.

30. Move from the Bottom of the Neck

Sitting, Standing or Lying: 30 seconds

Gently rest your hands on your face. Place your thumbs toward your ears and spread your fingers on your cheeks. Hold your head lightly.

Slowly make the movement of MMM across from left to right and right to left.

When making the movement, slowly lift and lower your forehead. Move so that the back of the head is closer and further from the ceiling.

Pay attention to your forehead during the movement. Pay attention to the movement at the base of the neck.

Make the movement small.

Rest.

Benefit:

Connect with the support of the hands touching the face. Reduce the strain to the upper part of the neck, jaw and face while easing the tension across the shoulders and down the arms using small movements of the neck

Observation:

Where does the movement happen in the neck?

What happens when you remove your hands from your cheeks and do the movement without support?

What happens if you hold the head tightly?
How large or small do you make the movement?

Caution:

Assess the speed and size of the movements.

How large are the muscles at the top of the neck along the spine and skull?

How large do the movements need to be to activate a muscle that is less than an inch long?

Rest often.

Pay attention to the origin of the movement when the forehead is the focus of attention.

31. Imagine

Standing, Sitting or Lying: 30-60 seconds

This is best when done often with attention and commitment to the time spent.

Find a quiet moment.

Take three "soft/belly" breaths to ready yourself (see no. 4, above).
Close your eyes if that is more comfortable or leave them open, your choice. Look out, soften your eyes, open your sight, and engage length and width to your view.

Open your mind.
Think of something important to you.

Use your senses.

Is this a visual picture? Is it a familiar scent or aroma? Do you hear tones or a song? Do you have a feeling or physical sense of something? All of these are correct.

Return to your original thought of something important.

What do you want?

Dream, set goals, expand your limitations and boundaries. Let go of the voice or image of limitation and past training which limited your receiving.

Make the image in your mind clear. Add details to bring life to the picture.

Rest.
Open your mind. Think of the thing that is important to you again.

What limits your picture?

Have you brought your sense of ownership to your picture? Is this where you desire to be in your life? Add what it takes to see yourself in the picture clearly.

How much do you want the picture to become real? How do you plan to receive the picture and integrate it as part of your life? What will you give to succeed in producing the picture?

Benefit:

Open possibilities for change, growth and to engage the brain in building future options. Imagination is the beginning of transformation. Find your new life.

Observation:

A clear picture helps define your reality.

Imagine yourself 1000 days into the future.

Imagine yourself being, doing, and participating in the picture you are creating. Get clear and creative.

Write your imagination pictures in a journal to check in the future and observe when you bring them into reality in your life.

Caution:

You might create what you picture.

You might limit your outcome.

You might find a new pathway.

You might find an escape from your daily life.

Sometimes a moment of escape is your outcome.

Imagine small and big. When you imagine small, make it as small as you are able. When you imagine big, make it as big as you are able. It takes time to learn and begin to receive. Move slowly in small ways with large vision.

Be prepared.

**Miracles happen to those
who imagine them.**

Just a Few of the Resources in America

- Brain Injury Association of America
- National Stroke Association
- American Heart Association
- AARP
- Wounded Warrior Project
- United States Department of Veterans Affairs
- American Medical Association
- American Academy of Neurology
- Academy of Nutrition and Dietetics
- National Institutes of Health
- National Family Caregivers Association
- American Physical Therapy Association
- American Occupational Therapy Association
- American Counseling Association
- Feldenkrais Guild of North America
- Foundation for Movement Intelligence
- International Feldenkrais Foundation
- Feldenkrais Resources
- Anat Baniel Method
- Center for Mind-Body Medicine
- Amen Clinics
- American Association of Naturopathic Physicians
- American Chinese Medicine Association
- MIT Dept. of Brain and Cognitive Sciences
- National Center for Complementary and Alternative Medicine
- The Organization for Brain Injury Professionals
- Head Injury Association
- American Speech-Language-Hearing Association
- American Thyroid Association

- National Association of Health Care Assistants
- National Collegiate Athletic Association
- American Massage Therapy Association
- American Bodywork & Massage Professionals
- Brain research and cognitive rehabilitation centers
- University neuroscience departments

ADD YOUR FAVORITES HERE

(Use this section here to write down anything you thought was most helpful)

Dedication and Huge Gratitude

Life is a process, not an event. There have been many people in my life who have been instrumental. My gratitude to each person listed and many more who were present throughout the phases of my learning process is boundless. Each member of my family participated in my journey with support, guidance, patience and love. This is not always a simple task.

I want to especially acknowledge my two amazing daughters, Kristina and Rachel. I dedicate a special thank you to my parents Mary O. and Allen K. Haller.

Thank you to every client who has given me the opportunity to share in the process of their session. From each of them I have received more clarity.

In addition, much gratitude to these people:

Susan Haller
Bob Haller and Wendy Seabloom
Mark and Linda Haller
Kathleen Lempka
Wendy Conner
Carl Longanecker
Marjorie Abrahamson
Dr. Rusheng Zheng
Brenda King
Maureen Lawler
Sheree Farber, PhD.
Nina Douglas
Michelle and Vern Cherwantanko, MD
Cheryl and Ales Koubik
Lauri and Mike Huston
Joe Pokora
Phoenix Alexander
Deanna Britton, PhC.

Leslee Dru Browning
Kelli Liddane

Feldenkrais Practitioners:

Moshe Feldenkrais, Dr.S.
Founder of the Feldenkrais Method

Ruthy Alon, GCFP
Jeff Haller PhD. GCFT
Mary Short Haller, GCFP
Elinor Silverstein, GCFP
Ellen Soloway, GCFP
Annie Thoe, GCFP
Olivia Cheever, EdD, GCFP
Denise Deig, MS, GCFP
Mariah Kruse, GCFP

To find a Guild Certified Feldenkrais Practitioner:
www.feldenkrais.com

Made in the USA
Monee, IL
29 October 2023